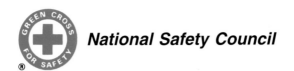

National Safety Council

First Aid
Pocket Guide

D0971133

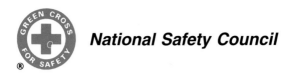

National Safety Council

First Aid
Pocket Guide

National Safety Council

and

Alton L. Thygerson

Technical Consultant
First Aid Institute
National Safety Council

Professor of Health Science
Brigham Young University

JONES AND BARTLETT PUBLISHERS

BOSTON   LONDON

Editorial, Sales, and Customer Service Offices
Jones and Bartlett Publishers
One Exeter Plaza
Boston, MA 02116
1-800-832-0034
617-859-3900

Jones and Bartlett Publishers International
7 Melrose Terrace
London W6 7RL
England

Library of Congress Cataloging-in Publication Data

Thygerson, Alton L.
     First aid pocket guide / Alton Thygerson.
       p. cm.
     Includes index.
     ISBN 0-86720-843-0
     1. First aid in illness and injury—Handbooks,
manuals, etc.
    I. Title.
    RC86.8.T49   1996   94-21045
    616.02 ' 52—dc20   CIP

Vice President and Publisher: Clayton Jones
Production Editor: Anne Noonan
Manufacturing Buyer: Dana L. Cerrito
Design: Glenna Collett
Editorial Production Service: York Production Services
Prepress: Lehigh Press Colortronics
Typesetting: York Graphic Services, Inc.
Cover Design: Marshall Henrichs

Printed in the United States of America
99 98 97 96 95   9 8 7 6 5 4 3 2 1

Contents

What Is First Aid? 1

Action at an Emergency 3

Approaching a Victim 3
Getting Help: Calling the EMS 4
Disease Precautions 5

Resuscitation 8

Adult Rescue Breathing and CPR 8
Choking 10

Finding Out What's Wrong 13

Primary Survey 13
Secondary Survey 16

**How to Treat Other
Life-Threatening Conditions** 18

Bleeding 18
Anaphylaxis (Severe Allergic Reaction) 20
Heart Attack 21
Heat Stroke 23
Chemical Exposure 24
Insulin Reaction 27

**Alphabetical Listing
of Emergencies** 29

Abdominal Injuries 29
Abdominal Pain 30

Amputations   30
Animal Bites   31
Ankle/Foot Injuries   33
Asthma   34
Back/Neck Injuries   35
Blisters   37
Broken Bone   39
Bruise   41
Burns, Heat/Thermal   42
Chest Injuries   46
Chest Pain   48
Dental/Mouth Injuries   49
Diabetic Emergencies   51
Dislocation   52
Electrocution   53
Eye Injuries   53
Fainting   57
Finger/Toe Injuries   58
Frostbite   61
Head Injuries   62
Heat Illnesses   66
Hyperventilation   68
Hypothermia   69
Muscle Injuries   72
Nose Injuries   72
Poison, Swallowed/Ingested   74
Poison Ivy, Oak, and Sumac   75
Seizures   78
Shock   79
Snakebites   81
Spider Bites and Scorpion Stings   84
Stings, Insect   87
Stroke   88
Substance Abuse   90
Tick Embedded   91
Wounds   92

Dressings and Bandages   95

Dressings   95
Bandages   96

Splinting Broken Bones and Dislocations 101

Moving a Victim 106

Shoulder Drag   106
One-Person Moves   106
Two-Person Moves   107

Appendix A: RICE Procedures for Muscle, Joint, and Bone Injuries 108

Appendix B: First Aid Supplies 111

Equipment   111
Bandage and Dressing Materials   112
Ointment and Topicals   113
Over-the-Counter Internal Medications   114
Miscellaneous   114

Introduction

This National Safety Council book arms you with immediate action steps for most injuries and sudden illnesses. Its size allows it to be a constant companion. Its conciseness allows a rapid review during an actual emergency and an occasional quick study to brush up on important "what to do" procedures. Its explanations are simple and easy to understand.

Since a physician or an ambulance is not usually needed, you can care for most injuries and sudden illnesses. The book tells when to seek medical attention and for life-threatening emergencies what to do until medical help arrives.

Because of the frequency of injuries and sudden illnesses, keep this book handy. Everyone will be faced with helping an injured or suddenly ill person.

Even though this book provides basic first aid information, it is not a substitute for a first aid course where skills can be developed. For such a course contact the National Safety Council (1-800-621-6244) for their nearest training agency or consult your telephone directory for a local National Safety Council chapter.

What Is First Aid?

All of us should be able to perform first aid because we will eventually find ourselves in a situation requiring it—either for another or for ourselves. The risk of injury while traveling, working, or playing is so great that most people sustain a significant injury at some time during their lives.

First aid is the immediate care given to the injured or suddenly ill person. First aid does *not* take the place of proper medical treatment. It consists only of furnishing temporary assistance until competent medical care, *if needed,* is obtained, or until the chance for recovery without medical care is assured. Most injuries and illnesses require only first aid care and not medical care.

The decision to help in most cases is strictly a moral one. However, you may find yourself in a situation in which the law requires you to give first aid (known as a "duty to act"). Such "duty" may be a part of your employment (i.e., lifeguard, park ranger, schoolteacher, athletic trainer, firefighter). Another "duty" that requires you to give first aid is when you have a preexisting relationship (i.e., parent, automobile driver) demanding you to be responsible for the victim.

Once you start giving first aid, you are legally bound to remain with the victim until you turn the victim's care over to an equally or better trained person or until the emergency medical service (EMS) arrives. For example, if you are doing CPR and an ambulance arrives with emergency medical technicians (EMT) capable of taking over, you may leave if you wish. But if a police car pulls up and the officer is unable to perform CPR, you cannot leave the victim without being guilty of abandonment. Abandonment in that situation means negligence, and negli-

gence can lead to an award of damages by a
court.

Fear of a lawsuit has made some people
wary of getting involved in emergency situations, even though Good Samaritan laws exist.
First aiders rarely are sued, and of those who
are, courts usually rule in their favor. Good
Samaritan laws cover medical personnel and
have been expanded in several states to include
laypersons serving as first aiders. These laws
say that if you help at an emergency when it is
not your "duty," you cannot be held guilty of
negligence unless what you did was so deviant
that it departed from all rational first aid guidelines.

Another concern is getting the victim's consent. Most of the time, consent is clear-cut—an
injured person does not refuse help or, if asked
by the first aider if help is needed, says yes. If a
situation involves a person needing but refusing
help, it is best to call the police because in most
locations the police can place a person in protective custody and require him or her to go to a
hospital. Another situation happens when a minor (person under the legal age) is injured and
parents or guardians are not readily available. It
is "implied" that a parent or guardian would give
consent for a first aider to render help without
their expressed consent.

Action at an Emergency

All of us will at some time have to make a decision whether or not to help another person. People react differently during an emergency. **The worst thing to do is nothing!**

APPROACHING A VICTIM

Scene Survey

Do a 10-second scene survey. As you approach an emergency scene, scan the area for immediate dangers to yourself or to the victim. For example, if an automobile accident has left the vehicle in the roadway, obstructing traffic, you have to consider whether you can safely go to that vehicle to help the victim. Or you might notice that gasoline is dripping from the gas tank and that the battery is shorted out and sparking: The car could explode at any moment. In such circumstances you should withdraw and get help before proceeding. It is not cowardly; it is merely realistic. Never make a rescue attempt that you have not been specifically trained to do. You cannot help another if you become a victim. Always ask: Is the scene safe to enter?

Another thing to do in the first 10 seconds is to determine the cause of the injury. For example, if a victim was thrown against a steering wheel, the emergency department physician must know this in order to check for liver, spleen, and cardiac injuries. Otherwise, the physician may never be able to recognize fully the extent of the injuries.

Determine how many people are injured. There may be more than one victim, so look around and ask about others involved.

GETTING HELP: CALLING THE EMS

When an emergency happens, generally you will
know it. You can tell by the type of injuries seen
or by the way the victim looks that it is time to
call the emergency medical service (EMS). Call
the EMS whenever the situation is more than
you can handle. Here is a list of some situations
when calling the EMS system is definitely the
right thing to do:

- Severe bleeding
- Drowning
- Electrocution
- Possible heart attack
- No breathing or difficulty breathing
- Choking
- Unconsciousness
- Poisoning
- Attempted suicide
- Some seizure cases—most do not require
  EMS assistance
- Critical burns
- Paralysis
- Possible spinal cord injury
- Imminent childbirth
- Cardiac arrest

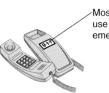

Most localities
use 911 for
emergencies.

When an
emergency oc-
curs, do not first
call your doctor,
the hospital, a
friend, relatives,
or neighbors for
help. First call the EMS (911 in most communities). Calling anyone else first will only waste
time.

If the situation is not an emergency, call
your doctor. However, if you are in any doubt as
to whether the situation is an emergency, call
the EMS.

How to Call the Emergency Medical Services (EMS) for Help

To receive emergency assistance of every kind in most communities, phone 911. Check to see if this is true in your community. An emergency telephone number should be listed on the inside front cover of all telephone directories. Keep these numbers near your telephones.

Be ready to give the EMS dispatcher the following information:

- *The victim's location.* Give address, names of intersecting streets or roads, and other landmarks if possible. This is the most important information you can give.
- *Your phone number and name.* This prevents false calls and allows the dispatch center to call back for additional information if needed.
- *What happened.* Tell the nature of the emergency (i.e., heart attack, drowning, etc.).
- *Number of persons* needing help and any special conditions.
- *Victim's condition* (i.e., conscious, breathing, etc.) and *what is being done* for the victim (i.e., rescue breathing, CPR, etc.).

Speak slowly and clearly. Always be the last to hang up the phone!

If you send someone else to call, have the person report back to you so that you can be sure the call was made.

DISEASE PRECAUTIONS

Bloodborne pathogens are disease-causing microorganisms that may be present in human blood. Two significant pathogens are hepatitis B virus (HBV) and human immunodeficiency virus (HIV). A number of bloodborne diseases other than HIV and HBV exist, such as hepatitis C, hepatitis D, and syphilis.

The HBV attacks the liver. HBV is very infectious and can cause:

- Active hepatitis B—a flulike illness that can last for months.
- A chronic carrier state—the person may have no symptoms but can pass HBV to others.
- Cirrhosis, liver cancer, and death.

Fortunately, vaccines are available to prevent HBV infection. Even if you are vaccinated against HBV, you must follow the "universal precautions"—treating all blood and certain human body fluids as if they are known to be infected with bloodborne pathogens.

HIV causes acquired immune deficiency syndrome (AIDS). HIV attacks the immune system, making the body less able to fight off infections. In most cases, these infections eventually prove fatal. At present there is no vaccine to prevent infection and no known cure for AIDS.

Use personal protective equipment whenever possible while giving first aid:

1. Keep open wounds covered with dressings to prevent contact with blood.

2. Use disposable latex gloves in every situation involving blood or other body fluids.

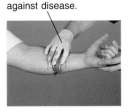

Disposable gloves protect against disease.

3. If disposable latex gloves are not available, use the most waterproof material available or extra gauze dressings to form a barrier.

4. Whenever possible, use a mouth-to-barrier device for protection when doing rescue

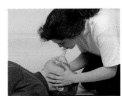

Mouth-to-barrier device with a one-way valve offers protection.

breathing. There may be blood in the victim's mouth.

After a person is exposed to blood or other body fluids:

1. Wash the exposed area immediately with soap and running water. Scrub vigorously with lots of lather.
2. Report the incident promptly, according to your workplace policy.
3. Get medical help, treatment, and counseling. If your workplace is covered by Occupational Safety and Health Administration's (OSHA) Bloodborne Standards, your employer must keep medical records confidential.
4. Ask about HBV globulin (HBIG) if you have not had the HBV vaccine. It can provide short-term protection. It is followed by vaccination against HBV.

Resuscitation

ADULT RESCUE BREATHING AND CPR

WHAT TO DO

If you see a motionless person:

1 **Check responsiveness** by tapping or gently shaking the victim.

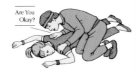

Are You Okay?

2 **Activate the EMS for help.** Activate by calling the local emergency telephone number, usually 911.

Most localities use 911 for emergencies.

3 **Roll person onto back.** If neck injury is suspected, move only if absolutely necessary and as a unit with the neck stabilized.

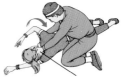

Gently roll victim's head and body together.

4 **Open airway.** Tilt the victim's head back by lifting the chin gently with one hand while pushing down on the forehead with the other hand.

If a neck injury is suspected, do not move the victim's head or neck. First try lifting chin without tilting the head back. If breaths do not go in, gently and slowly bend head back until breaths go in.

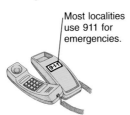

5 Check for breathing (take 3 to 5 seconds). Put your ear over the victim's mouth and nose while keeping the airway open. Look at the victim's chest to check for a rise and fall; listen and feel for breathing.

6 Give two slow breaths. While using the head-tilt/chin-lift to keep airway open, pinch the nose shut. Take a deep breath and seal your lips tightly around the victim's mouth. Give 2 slow breaths (1 1/2 to 2 seconds) while pausing between them to take a breath. Watch chest rise to see if breaths go in.

If neither of these 2 breaths went in, retilt the head and try 2 more breaths. If still unsuccessful, suspect choking and use appropriate procedures, explained later. (Give 5 abdominal thrusts; perform tongue-jaw lift followed by a finger sweep; give 2 more breaths; retilt and give 2 more. Repeat if necessary.)

7 Check for pulse (take 5 to 10 seconds). While keeping victim's head tilted back, place fingers on the Adam's apple and then slide these fingers down into the groove of the neck on the side closest to you.

8 Perform rescue procedures based on what you found: *If there is a pulse,* give rescue breaths every 5 to 6 seconds. Every minute stop and check the pulse.

If there is no pulse, give CPR. Find the proper hand position by sliding your fingers up the ribcage edge to the notch where the ribs meet the breastbone. Place your middle finger in the notch with your index finger next to it. Put heel of other hand on breastbone next to index finger. Remove hand from the notch, put it on top of hand on the chest, and interlace your fingers. Keep your fingers up off the victim's chest.

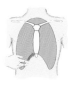

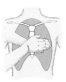

Give 15 compressions by placing your shoulders directly over your hands on the chest, keeping arms straight and elbows locked, pushing breastbone straight down 1 1/2 to 2 inches. Count as you push down: "one and, two and, three and, four and, five and, six and, seven and, . . . , fifteen and." Follow compressions with 2 slow breaths.

Continue cycles of 15 compressions to 2 breaths. Recheck the pulse every few minutes. After a pulse check, restart CPR with chest compressions.

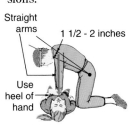

Straight arms
1 1/2 - 2 inches
Use heel of hand

Continue until victim is revived, you are relieved by trained help, or you are completely exhausted.

CHOKING

Choking occurs when the upper airway becomes blocked and the victim cannot breathe.

WHAT TO DO

If adult is conscious and cannot speak, breathe, or cough:

1 Give up to five abdominal thrusts. Stand behind victim; wrap your arms around victim's waist. Make fist with one hand and place it just above victim's navel and well below the tip of the breastbone with the knuckles up. Grasp fist with your other hand.

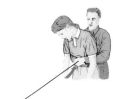

Press fist with quick upward thrusts

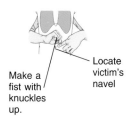

Make a fist with knuckles up.

Locate victim's navel

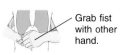

Grab fist with other hand.

Press fist into victim's abdomen with 5 quick, upward thrusts. Each thrust should be a separate and distinct effort to dislodge the object. After every 5 abdominal thrusts, check the victim and your technique.

2 Repeat cycles of up to five abdominal thrusts until victim coughs up object, starts to breathe, or coughs forcefully, until you are relieved by the EMS or other trained person, or until the victim becomes unconscious (then use methods for unconscious victim).

For a late-stage pregnant woman or obese person, stand behind the victim, place your arms under the victim's armpits, and encircle the chest. Place a fist on the middle of the victim's breastbone with your knuckles up. Grasp your fist with your other hand and press backward with up to 5 thrusts.

*If adult is unconscious and 2 breaths have not
gone in, and after retilting the head 2 more
breaths have not gone in:*

**1 Give up to 5
abdominal thrusts.**
Straddle victim's
thighs, put heel of one
hand against middle of
victim's abdomen
slightly above navel
and well below breast-
bone's notch (keep fin-
gers pointing toward
victim's head). Put
other hand directly on
top of the first hand.
Push inward and up-
ward using both hands
with up to 5 quick ab-
dominal thrusts. Each
thrust should be a dis-
tinct attempt to dis-
lodge the object.

Fingers point
toward head.

Press inward and upward
using both hands.

Note: For a late-stage
pregnant woman or
obese person, consider
using chest thrusts.

**2 Perform finger
sweep.** Use your
thumb and fingers to
grasp victim's jaw and
tongue and lift upward

to pull tongue away
from back of throat.

Grasp victim's
jaw and tongue.

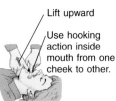

Lift upward

Use hooking
action inside
mouth from one
cheek to other.

With the index finger
of your other hand,
slide finger down
along the inside of one
cheek, deeply into
mouth, and use a
hooking action across
to other cheek to dis-
lodge foreign object. If
object comes within
reach, grab and re-
move it.

If the airway re-
mains blocked, rotate
through cycles of 2
rescue breaths, retilt
head and give 2 more
breaths, perform up to
5 abdominal thrusts,
and perform finger
sweeps until object is
removed or the EMS
replaces you.

Finding Out What's Wrong

During emergency situations when panic exists, knowing what to do and what not to do can be vital. You cannot help if you do not know what is wrong. Presented here is a method that can be recalled during those hectic, panicky, emergency situations when you may be wondering what to do first.

Checking a victim is divided into two parts:

- Primary survey for life-threatening conditions
- Secondary survey for nonemergency conditions

After determining if the situation is safe to proceed (see page 3), you can do a primary survey. Make all checks while kneeling close to the victim. If two or more people are injured, go to the quiet one first because the airway may not be open and he or she may not be breathing or have a pulse. The victim who is talking, crying, or yelling obviously is breathing.

Most of the first aid you give will not require a complete victim assessment because the injuries will be of the "band-aid" type.

PRIMARY SURVEY

The *primary survey* finds and corrects life-threatening conditions. Most primary surveys will be quickly completed because most injured victims you see won't have life-threatening conditions. A previous section on resuscitation (see page 8) gives in detail the first parts of a primary survey: the ABCs.

If the primary survey uncovers any problems, such as no breathing or massive bleeding,

you must attend to them immediately before proceeding with the rest of the assessment.

The primary survey steps can be remembered by using the acronym **ABCHs:**

A—Airway Open? If the victim is talking or is
conscious, the airway is open. If the victim is
unconscious, open the airway with the head-
tilt/chin-lift method unless a neck injury is
suspected, in which case you use other methods. See page 8 for details.

B—Breathing? Conscious people are breathing.
However, note any breathing difficulties or unusual breathing sounds. If the victim is unconscious, keep the airway open and look for the
chest to rise and fall, listen for breathing, and
feel for air coming out of the victim's nose and
mouth. See page 8 for details.

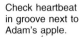
Check heartbeat
in groove next to
Adam's apple.

C—Circulation? Check circulation by feeling for a pulse at
the side of the neck
(carotid artery). If a
pulse is absent, CPR is
required. See page 9 for
details.

H—Hemorrhage? Check
for severe bleeding by
looking over the entire
body for blood (blood-
soaked clothing and/or
blood pooling on the
floor or the ground).
Bleeding requires the
application of direct

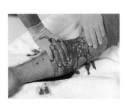

pressure over the spot that is bleeding. Try to
avoid contact with the victim's blood by using
disposable latex gloves or extra layers of cloth
or dressings. See page 5 for details.

s—Spinal Cord Injury? Check for a spinal cord
injury, especially when any event such as a fall
or motor vehicle crash occurs that could pro-

duce spine injury. Assume a victim with a head injury has a spine injury until proven otherwise. A test of the spinal cord is the Babinski test: Stroke the bottom of the foot firmly toward the big toe with a key or similar sharp object. The big toe goes down in normal adults (except in infants). If the toe goes up, suspect a spinal or brain injury. If a spine injury is suspected, do not move the victim's head or neck and keep it stable with your hands (see page 35).

Checking for Spinal Cord Injuries

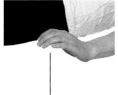

Victim wiggles fingers.

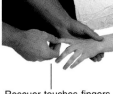

Rescuer touches fingers.

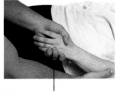

Victim squeezes rescuer's hand.

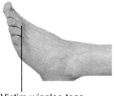

Victim wiggles toes.

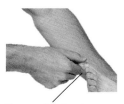

Rescuer touches toes.

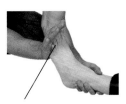

Victim pushes foot against rescuer's hand.

Clothing may be hiding an injury. How much clothing should be removed varies, depending on what conditions or injuries are found. The general rule is to remove as much clothing as necessary to determine the presence or absence of a condition or injury. Avoid hypothermia: Most injured victims will be susceptible. If clothing needs to be removed which may prove embarrassing to the victim and/or bystanders, explain what you intend to do and why.

SECONDARY SURVEY

After completing the primary survey and attending to any life-threatening problems it uncovers, make a systematic victim assessment called the *secondary survey.* This survey will discover injuries and/or conditions that do not pose an immediate threat to life, but may do so if they remain undetected and uncorrected. Even minor injuries need treatment, but must first be found.

The secondary survey steps can be remembered by using the mnemonic **CH^{2}ECK:**

C—Chief Complaint. This is the victim's answer when you ask, "What's wrong?" or "Where do you hurt?"

H^2—History. Try to find out two things:

1. What caused the injury or condition.
2. What medical problems does the victim have that may be causing the condition or information about which should be passed on to the EMS system, such as (a) allergies, (b) medications, and (c) past health problems.

E—Exact Location. Gently touch, feel, or probe the injury site for any obvious or unusual deformity. This "looking and feeling" survey can be remembered by using look, ask, feel (**LAF**) as a reminder of how to examine a victim:

- **L**—**L**ook for injuries such as blood, deformity, swelling.
- **A**—**A**sk the victim about pain.
- **F**—**F**eel for tenderness, swelling, deformity.

C—**C**ompare. If possible, compare the injured area with the same area on the opposite side of the body to determine anything unusual.

K—**K**eep Checking. Keep checking the ABCHs and keep a written record of what you find. This will help a physician, should one be needed, with a later diagnosis.

Once the secondary survey is completed you will know what is wrong. You can then give better first aid.

Medical Alert Tag

A medical alert emblem tag is worn as a necklace or as a bracelet to attract attention in an emergency situation. These tags contain the wearer's medical problem(s) and a 24-hour telephone number to call in case of an emergency that offers access to the victim's medical history plus names of doctors and close relatives. Necklaces and bracelets are durable,

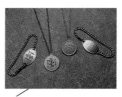

Medical alert tags (front)

Medical problem on back.

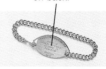

instantly recognizable, and less likely than cards to be separated from the victim in an emergency.

How to Treat Other Life-Threatening Conditions

BLEEDING

WHAT TO DO

1 Protect yourself against disease. Wear disposable latex gloves. If gloves are unavailable, use several layers of gauze pads or cloth, plastic wrap or bag, or have the victim apply pressure with his or her hand.

2 Cover the entire wound with a gauze pad or clean cloth and press firmly with your fingers or palm.

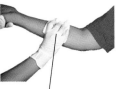

Direct pressure stops most bleeding. Place sterile gauze pad or clean cloth over wound. Wear disposable gloves. If bleeding does not stop in 10 minutes, press harder over a wider area.

3 If bleeding does not stop in 10 minutes, the pressure may be too light or in the wrong location. Press harder over a wider area for another 10 minutes. If the bleeding is from an arm or leg, while pressing over the wound, raise the bleeding site above the heart's level. Elevation alone will not stop bleeding.

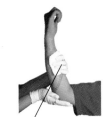

If bleeding persists, use elevation to help reduce blood flow. It must be combined with direct pressure over the wound.

DO NOT remove a blood-soaked dressing. Place another dressing on top and keep pressing.

4 If bleeding still continues, press with your fingers over a pressure point to slow the flow of blood while continuing to apply pressure over the wound. These pressure points are on the upper inside arm (brachial) and near the groin (femoral).

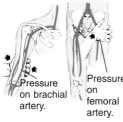

Pressure on brachial artery.

Pressure on femoral artery.

5 After the bleeding stops, or if you need to be free to care for other injuries and/or victims, apply a pressure bandage on the wound. Wrap a roller gauze bandage tightly over the dressing and above and below the wound site. DO NOT apply a pressure bandage so tight that it cuts off circulation. DO NOT use a tourniquet—they are rarely needed, and the victim risks losing the arm or leg.

6 Treat for shock by raising the legs 8 to 12 inches and covering the victim with a coat or blanket to keep the victim warm.

7 When direct pressure cannot be applied (i.e., protruding bone, skull fracture, embedded object), use a doughnut-shaped (ring) pad to control bleeding.

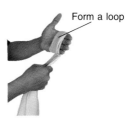

Form a loop

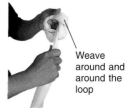

Weave around and around the loop

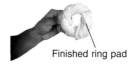

Finished ring pad

Make a ring pad by using a narrow bandage (roller or cravat) to form a loop around one hand by wrapping one end of the bandage several times around your four fingers. Pass the other end through the loop and wrap it around and around until the entire bandage is used and a ring is made.

8 Care for the wound (see page 92).

9 Seek medical attention if you can not stop the bleeding.

Internal Bleeding

If you suspect internal bleeding (i.e., painful abdomen, blood in vomit or stool—these and others may take days to appear):

1 Check the ABCHs.

2 Expect vomiting. Keep the victim lying on his or her left side to help prevent vomiting, for drainage, and to protect the lungs from inhaling the vomit. DO NOT give victim anything to eat or drink.

3 If the victim is not vomiting, raise the legs 8 to 12 inches and cover the victim with a coat or blanket. See page 80 for when to use other body positions.

4 Seek medical attention immediately.

ANAPHYLAXIS (SEVERE ALLERGIC REACTION)

Allergic reactions range from mild to serious. Allergic reactions that are sudden and massive are known as anaphylaxis. Such reactions can be caused by an insect sting, a particular food or food additive, or a particular drug. If untreated, anaphylaxis can be fatal within 5 to 30 minutes. *It is life-threatening!*

WHAT TO LOOK FOR

- Sneezing, coughing, or wheezing
- Shortness of breath

- Tightness and swelling in the throat
- Tightness in the chest
- Severe itching, burning, rash, or hives on the skin
- Swelling of face, tongue, mouth
- Blue around lips and mouth
- Dizziness and weakness
- Nausea and vomiting
- Unconsciousness

WHAT TO DO

1 Check the ABCs.

2 Epinephrine is the only lifesaving treatment for anaphylaxis. If the victim has his or her own physician-prescribed epinephrine kit, help the victim to use it. First aiders do not have access to epinephrine except through a victim's kit. Follow the kit's instructions.

3 Seek medical at-

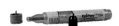

Doctor prescribed pre-loaded epinephrine auto-injector.

tention immediately.

4 Keep a conscious victim sitting up to help breathing; place an unconscious victim in the "recovery position" (on the side).

5 Keep checking the ABCs.

HEART ATTACK

A heart attack happens when the blood supply to part of the heart muscle is severely reduced or stopped.

WHAT TO LOOK FOR

The American Heart Association lists these as possible signs and symptoms of a heart attack:

- Pressure, squeezing, or pain in the center of the chest that lasts more than a few minutes, or goes away and comes back
- Pain spreading to the shoulders, neck, or arms
- Chest discomfort with lightheadedness, fainting, sweating, nausea, or shortness of breath

Not all of these warning signs occur in every heart attack. It is difficult to determine heart attacks. Expect someone with chest discomfort to deny the possibility of something as serious as a heart attack. Don't take "no" for an answer. Insist on taking prompt action.

WHAT TO DO

1 Call the EMS or get to the nearest hospital emergency department that offers 24-hour emergency cardiac care.

2 Check the ABCs. If necessary, give CPR (see page 8) if you are properly trained.

3 Help the victim to the least painful position—usually sitting with legs up and bent at the knees. Loosen clothing around the neck and midriff. Be calm and reassuring.

4 Determine if the victim has physician-prescribed medicine for angina. If the victim is conscious, help him or her take it. (Usually nitroglycerin comes as tablets, a spray to be applied under the tongue, or in ointment that is placed on the skin.)

Help the victim into a relaxed position to ease strain on the heart.

Half sitting position.

Place padding under knees.

Support back.

Knees bent.

HEAT STROKE

Heat stroke's high body temperature can damage tissues and organs throughout the body. Untreated victims always die.

WHAT TO LOOK FOR

A victim who has been in a hot environment who shows:

- Hot skin with a high body temperature
- Altered mental status (i.e., confusion, disorientation, agitation, bizarre behavior, seizures, unconsciousness)
- Rapid breathing and pulse
- Dry or wet skin. Dry skin happens in most victims; however, sweating may be seen in 50 percent of exertional heat stroke victims (usually healthy people working or playing in a hot environment).

WHAT TO DO

1 Check and recheck the ABCs.

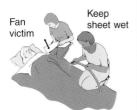

Fan victim

Keep sheet wet

2 Move the victim to a cool place. Remove clothing; lightweight cotton clothing can be left in place.

3 Cool the victim by any available means as fast as possible.

If in low humidity (less than 75 percent), use the evaporation method by either:

- Spraying or pouring water on the victim and at the same time vigorously fanning the victim, or
- Covering victim with wet sheet or similar cotton cloth, keeping it wet, and fanning the victim.

If in high humidity (greater than 75 percent), the evaporation method does not work very well. Place ice packs on areas with abundant blood supply (i.e., neck, armpits, groin).

Stop cooling when there is an improvement in consciousness and mental status. If you have a thermometer, stop when the temperature reaches 102° F. DO NOT try to reduce body temperature by using aspirin or acetaminophen or sponging with alcohol.

4 Keep head and shoulders slightly elevated.

5 If seizures occur, treat the victim (see page 78).

6 Seek medical attention immediately.

CHEMICAL EXPOSURE

A caustic or corrosive substance can damage tissue within 1 to 5 minutes, so speed in removing the chemical is vital.

WHAT TO DO

Seek medical attention immediately for all chemical exposures.

If a chemical is on the skin: A caustic or corrosive substance continues to burn as long as it stays in contact with the skin. Alkali burns (i.e., from drain cleaners) are more serious than acid burns (i.e., from battery acid) because they penetrate deeper and remain active longer.

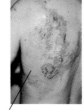

Chemical burn: sulfuric acid

1 Immediately flush the chemical with large amounts of water (i.e., hose, shower, faucet, or bucket).

DO NOT use

strong pressure. Dry powder chemicals should be brushed from the skin before flushing

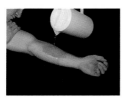

2   Remove the victim's contaminated

clothing while flushing with water.

3   Flush for 15 to 20 minutes or even longer. Let the victim wash with a mild soap before a final rinse.

4   Cover the affected skin with a dry, sterile dressing, or, for large areas, use a clean sheet.

If a chemical is in an eye:

1   Use your fingers to keep the eye open as wide as possible.

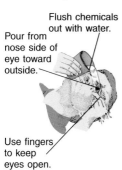

Pour from nose side of eye toward outside.

Flush chemicals out with water.

Use fingers to keep eyes open.

2   Flush the eye with water immediately. If possible, use warm water. If water is not available, use any nonirritating liq-

uid such as milk or soda pop.

3   Hold the head under a faucet or pour water into the eye from any clean container for at least 15 to 20 minutes, continuously and gently.

- Irrigate from the nose side of the eye toward the outside to avoid flushing material into the other eye.

- Tell the victim to roll his or her eyeball as much as

possible to wash out the eye.

4 Loosely bandage both eyes with cold, wet dressings.

If a caustic or corrosive chemical was swallowed:

1 Give water or milk (see page 74).

If a chemical was breathed (inhaled):

WHAT TO LOOK FOR

It is difficult to tell if a victim has been "gassed." Sometimes, a complaint of having the "flu" is really a symptom of contact with a toxic gas. Although many symptoms resemble flu, there are differences. For example, carbon monoxide poisoning does not produce low-grade fever, generalized aching, or lymph node involvement. Inhaled poison symptoms will:
- Come and go
- Worsen or improve in certain places or at certain times of the day
- Involve others in the vicinity with similar symptoms
- Cause pets to seem ill

Inhaled poisoning signs and symptoms are:
- Headache
- Ringing in the ears (tinnitus)
- Chest pain (angina)
- Muscle weakness
- Nausea and vomiting
- Dizziness and visual changes (blurred or double vision)
- Unconsciousness
- Breathing and cardiac arrest

WHAT TO DO

1 Remove the victim from the toxic environment and into fresh air immediately.

2 Check and recheck the ABCs.

3 Seek medical attention immediately.

INSULIN REACTION

An insulin reaction happens when a person with diabetes takes too much insulin or eats too little food after taking insulin or other diabetes medications.

WHAT TO LOOK FOR

An insulin reaction can be difficult to recognize and can be confused with other medical conditions. Look for a medical alert tag. See page 51 for Diabetic Coma, another diabetic emergency.

The American Diabetes Association lists the following signs and symptoms of low blood sugar (insulin reaction or hypoglycemia):

- Sudden onset
- Staggering, poor coordination
- Anger, bad temper
- Pale color
- Confusion, disorientation
- Sudden hunger
- Excessive sweating
- Trembling
- Eventual unconsciousness

WHAT TO DO

If the victim is conscious:

1 Provide sugar (i.e., sugar cube, soda drink, candy, or fruit juice). DO NOT use diet drinks—they do not contain sugar.

2 If the person is not better in 10 to 15 minutes, seek medical attention immediately.

If the victim is unconscious:

1 Check the ABCs.

2 Seek medical attention immediately.

3 Treat any seizures (see page 78).

4 If you are in a remote setting or if medical attention is some distance away, place sugar under the victim's tongue to dissolve.

Alphabetical Listing of Emergencies

ABDOMINAL INJURIES

Abdominal injuries have two parts: what you see (external) and what you do not see (internal).

Seek medical attention for all abdominal injuries.

Blow to the Abdomen

Place the victim on the left side in a comfortable position. DO NOT give the victim any food or drink.

Penetrating Wound

Stabilize the object in place and control bleeding by using bulky dressings around it. DO NOT remove the object.

Protruding Organs

1 DO NOT try to reinsert protruding organs inside the abdomen because this introduces infection and could damage the intestines.

2 Cover protruding organs with a sterile dressing or clean cloth. DO NOT cover the organs with any material that clings or disintegrates when wet.

3 Pour drinkable water on the dressing to keep the protruding organ from drying out.

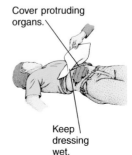

Cover protruding organs.

Keep dressing wet.

ABDOMINAL PAIN

Though many disorders cause abdominal pain, first aid is the same. Some conditions can be life-threatening and will require surgery.

WHAT TO DO

1 DO NOT allow the victim to eat or drink.

2 DO NOT give the victim laxatives, enemas, or pain medications.

3 If there is burning pain, give an antacid.

4 Keep the victim in a comfortable position, usually with knees bent. If vomiting is expected keep the victim on the left side.

5 Seek medical attention if any of these accompany the abdominal pain:

- Severe pain
- Pain lasts more than 12 hours.
- Abdominal injury
- Bloody stool
- Fever
- Pregnant woman

AMPUTATIONS

An amputation is a complete cutting off of a body part (i.e., finger, ear, leg). Surgical techniques can sometimes reattach amputated parts so they function normally or nearly normal.

WHAT TO DO

1 Check the ABCHs (see page 14) and control bleeding (see page 18).

2 Treat for shock (see page 79).

3 Find and save the amputated part, and whenever possible keep it with the victim. Let the physician decide if the part can be saved.

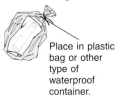

Wrap amputated body part in dry, sterile gauze.

Place in plastic bag or other type of waterproof container.

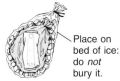

Place on bed of ice: do *not* bury it.

4 To care for an amputated part:

- Rinse the part with clean water to remove any debris—do not scrub.
- Wrap the amputated part with a dry sterile gauze or other available clean cloth. A wet wrapping can cause waterlogging and tissue softening. When these occur, the part is more difficult to reattach.
- Put the wrapped amputated part in a plastic bag or waterproof container (i.e., cup, pot).
- Place the bag or container with the wrapped part on a bed of ice. DO NOT bury an amputated part in ice. Reattaching frostbitten parts is usually unsuccessful.

5 Seek medical attention immediately.

DO NOT cut a small skin "bridge," tendon, or partially attached part attaching the injured part to the rest of the body. Reposition the part in the normal position, wrap the part in a dry sterile dressing or clean cloth, and place an ice pack on it.

ANIMAL BITES

WHAT TO DO

1 If the wound is not bleeding heavily, wash it with soap and water for 5 to 10 minutes. DO NOT scrub; scrubbing bruises tissue. Allow the wound to bleed a little to help remove bacteria left in the tissues.

Dog bite

2 Rinse the wound with running water under pressure.

3 Control bleeding (see page 18).

4 Cover with a sterile dressing. DO NOT seal the wound with tape or butterfly bandages. This traps bacteria in the wound and increases the chance of infection.

5 Seek medical attention for further wound cleaning, tetanus shot, and stitches to close the wound.

Rabies

A virus found in warm-blooded animals causes rabies and spreads from one animal to another, usually through a bite or by licking involving saliva from

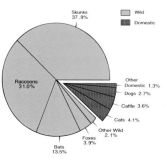

Cases of Rabies in Animals

an infected animal. Ninety-six percent of the rabies cases in the United States come from skunks, raccoons, and bats.

WHAT TO DO

1 Try to locate the animal's owner or, in the case of a wild animal, find its location.

2 Call the police or animal control officer to capture the animal for observation. When

the animal cannot be found or identified, the bitten victim must usually go through a series of rabies shots (vaccinations).

3 DO NOT go near or try to capture the

A

animal yourself. DO NOT kill the animal. If it is killed, protect the head and brain from damage so they can be examined for rabies. If it is dead, transport the animal intact to prevent exposure to the potentially infected tissues or saliva. If necessary, the animal's remains can be refrigerated (avoid freezing).

Human Bites

After dogs and cats, the animal most likely to bite humans is another human. Human bites can cause a very severe injury. The human mouth contains a wide range of bacteria, and the chance of infection is greater from a human bite than from bites of other warm-blooded animals. Care for a human bite is the same as for an animal bite.

ANKLE/FOOT INJURIES

A

WHAT TO LOOK FOR

It is difficult to tell the difference between a severely sprained ankle and a broken one. Assume it is broken until you can get the advice of a physician. The following suggestions, although not 100 percent accurate, may help you determine whether the injury is a sprain or a fracture:

1. Press along the bones. Pain and tenderness over the bones at either the (a) back edge or tip of either of the ankle knob bones (malleolus bones) or (b) midfoot's outside bone or on the inside may indicate a broken bone.
2. Ask the victim, "Did you try standing on it?" Putting some weight on the ankle may hurt a little, but if the victim is able to do that and take four or more steps, most likely the ankle is sprained. If it is broken, the victim will not want to put any weight on it, and if walking is tried, no more than four steps will be taken.

WHAT TO DO

1 Take the shoe off to check and care for the injury.

2 Check the foot's **CSM** (circulation, sensation, movement)—see page 40.

3 Use the **RICE** procedures (see page 108). Every minute the RICE procedure is delayed can add an hour to healing. The goal of RICE is to limit swelling.

ASTHMA

People with asthma have acute episodes (some people say "attack" or "flare") when the air passages in their lungs get narrower and breathing becomes more difficult. Some people develop asthma in very cold weather—called "cold allergy." Others have it during strenuous exertion—called exercise-induced asthma. Other triggers of asthma include allergies; air pollution; infections; emotions such as anger, crying, and laughing too hard; and smoke.

WHAT TO LOOK FOR

Asthma varies a great deal from one person to another, ranging from mild to severe, and can be life-threatening. The episodes can come only occasionally or often. Look for:

- Coughing
- Blue skin
- Victim unable to speak in complete sentences without pausing for breath
- Nostrils flaring with each breath
- Wheezing—high-pitched whistling sound during breathing

WHAT TO DO

1 The victim should rest and take physician-prescribed asthma medicines.

2 Help the victim into a comfortable

breathing position, which is usually sitting upright.

3 In case of a severe, prolonged episode, seek medical attention immediately.

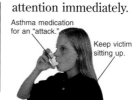

Asthma medication for an "attack."

Keep victim sitting up.

BACK/NECK INJURIES

All injured, unconscious victims should be treated as though they have a spinal injury. Suspect a spinal injury in all victims sustaining injuries from falls, diving accidents, or motor vehicle crashes.

WHAT TO LOOK FOR

- Head injury (15 to 20 percent of victims of head injury also have a spine injury)
- Painful movement of arms and/or legs
- Numbness, tingling, weakness, or burning sensation in arms or legs
- Loss of bowel or bladder control
- Paralysis to arms and/or legs
- Deformity; odd-looking angle of the victim's head and neck
- Test the spinal cord by stroking the bottom of the foot firmly toward the big toe with a key or similar sharp object (known as the Babinski test). It is normal if the big toe goes down (but not in infants). With spinal cord or brain injury, an adult's toe will go up.

Ask a conscious victim these questions:

- "Is there pain? "Neck injuries radiate pain to the arms; upper-back injuries radiate pain around the ribs; lower-back injuries usually radiate pain down the legs. Often the victim describes the pain as "electric."
- "Can you move your feet?" Ask the victim to move his or her foot against your hand. If the victim cannot perform this movement or if the

B

movement is extremely weak against your hand, the victim may have injured the spinal cord.

- "Can you move your fingers?" Moving the fingers is a sign that nerve pathways are intact. Ask the victim to grip your hand. A strong grip indicates that a spinal cord injury is unlikely.

Checking for Spinal Cord Injuries

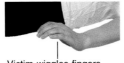

Victim wiggles fingers.

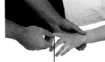

Rescuer touches fingers.

Victim squeezes rescuer's hand.

Victim wiggles toes.

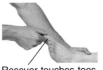

Rescuer touches toes.

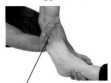

Victim pushes foot against rescuer's hand.

For an unconscious victim:

- Test responses by pinching the victim's hands (either palm or back) and foot (sole or top of the bare foot). No reaction could mean spinal cord damage. Also use the Babinski test described above and shown below.

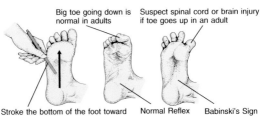

Big toe going down is normal in adults

Suspect spinal cord or brain injury if toe goes up in an adult

Stroke the bottom of the foot toward big toe with a blunt object.

Normal Reflex

Babinski's Sign Present

B

WHAT TO DO

1 Check and recheck the ABCHs. Use the proper method in a non-breathing victim because of possible damage to the spinal cord (see page 8).

2 Call the EMS.

3 Keep the victim in the position found.

4 Stabilize the victim against any movement.

If victim is lying down:

- Grasp the victim's collarbone (clavicle) and shoulder (trapezius) muscle, cradle the head between the inside of your forearms, and

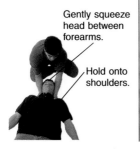

Gently squeeze head between forearms.

Hold onto shoulders.

hold the head and neck still until the EMS arrives. Tell the victim not to move.

If you are tired from holding the head in place and/or other victims need help:

- Place heavy objects on either side of the head to prevent it moving from side to side.

If the victim is seated upright:

- Support the head. DO NOT move the victim—wait for the EMS.

If the victim is in water (i.e., pool, lake):

- DO NOT remove a victim from water unless you are trained and have a long backboard. Float the victim to the surface and near the water's edge. Stabilize the neck and body against movement. Wait for the EMS.

B

BLISTERS

A blister is a collection of fluid in a "bubble" under the outer layer of skin. It results from excessive rubbing or friction. (This section does not apply to blisters from burns, frostbite, or contact with a poisonous plant.)

WHAT TO DO

If area on skin becomes a "hot spot" (painful, red area):

1 Apply a piece of smooth tape or silver aluminum duct tape, or

2 Cover it with Spenco Second Skin™ (absorbs friction) or a doughnut-shaped moleskin secured by tape.

If blister on foot is unbroken and not very painful:

1 Cut doughnut shaped holes in several gauze pads, moleskin, or molefoam to fit around the blister.

2 Place several layers of gauze pads or moleskin with holes around blister.

3 Tape an uncut gauze pad over doughnut-shaped gauze pads or moleskin.

Or cover blister with Spenco Second Skin™.

If blister on foot is broken, or if a very painful unbroken blister affects walking/running:

1 Clean the area with soap and water.

2 Drain all fluid from blister by making several small holes at the base of the blister with a sterilized needle. Press the fluid out. Do not remove the blister's roof unless it is torn.

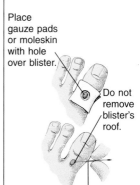

Place gauze pads or moleskin with hole over blister.

Do not remove blister's roof.

Painful blister can be drained by making small hole with sterilized needle.

Cut holes in several gauze pads or moleskin.

3 Apply antibiotic ointment.

4 Use procedures listed above for treating an unbroken blister.

5 Change dressing daily and check daily for infection (redness and pus). Seek medical attention if infection develops.

BROKEN BONE

There is no sure way to tell if a bone is broken except by x-ray examination. Therefore, when in doubt, treat victim as if the bone were broken.

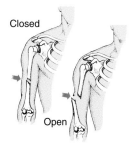

Closed

Open

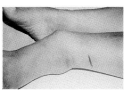

Closed fracture: severe deformity

B

WHAT TO DO

1 Treat the victim for shock (see page 79).

2 Gently remove clothing covering the injured area. DO NOT move the injured area unless necessary.

3 Use **LAF** (look, ask, feel) to examine the area:

L—: **L**ook at the injured area for swelling or deformity; compare the injured area to the same uninjured area on the other side of victim's body.

A—: **A**sk the victim to rate the pain; ask how the injury happened; and ask if the victim can use the injured part.

F—: area tender when **F**elt

4 Check **c**irculation and nerves by using

CSM: **c**irculation, **s**ensation, **m**ovement. Check the **CSM** before and after applying a splint.

- **C**—Check **C**irculation in an injured extremity by using the radial pulse at the wrist for an arm injury or the posterior ankle pulse (located between the inside ankle bone and achilles tendon) for a leg injury.
- **S**—Check **S**ensation by lightly touching the victim's toes or fingers and asking the victim to report when your touch is felt to check for nerve damage.
- **M**—**M**ovement is to the ability to wiggle the toes or fingers to check for nerve damage.

5 Stabilize the injured part in place.

- Most broken bones are minor, and the part usually does not need straightening. If you are unsure what the part should look like, check the undamaged part. If the victim shows increased pain or if you feel resistance, stop your attempts to straighten, and splint the extremity as it is.
- Try to straighten any arm or leg with no **CSM** to restore blood flow. If pulse is not restored, seek immediate medical attention. DO NOT straighten broken bones involving the spine, shoulder, elbow, wrist, or knee because of the possibility of damaging nerves and arteries near these joints.
- Many different materials can be used as splints. Examples are folded newspapers, cardboard, wood board, pillow, or the victim's body by tying the injured part to an uninjured adjacent part.
- Apply a splint to stabilize the joint above and the joint below the injury

site. For example, a fractured forearm bone requires stabilizing the wrist and the elbow. If you stabilize the wrist only, the forearm bone can still move whenever the elbow turns.

- For an injured joint, stabilize the bones above and below the joint.
- When possible, place splint materials on both sides of the injured part ("sandwich splint") to prevent bones from rotating.

BRUISE

A bruise (contusion) results when a blunt object strikes the body and the small blood vessels beneath the skin are broken. The skin is not broken, and no blood can be seen on the skin's surface. A bruise is discolored, swollen, and painful, and may limit use of a body part.

WHAT TO DO

1 Apply an ice pack for 20 minutes. DO NOT put ice directly on the skin. Protect the victim's skin from frostbite by placing a wet cloth between the ice and the skin. The wet cloth transfers cold better than a dry one, which insulates.

2 If an arm or leg is involved, apply an elastic bandage with several gauze pads over the area and under the bandage.

3 Check for a possible fracture.

4 Keep an injured arm or leg, if it is not broken, above the victim's heart level to decrease pain and swelling.

5 Seek medical attention for:

- bruises that show up for no apparent reason
- suspected broken bone
- suspected internal bleeding

BURNS, HEAT/THERMAL

WHAT TO DO

1 Stop the burning (best done with water). DO NOT pull stuck clothing; cut around it.

2 Check the ABCs.

3 Determine the depth of the burn. This can be difficult even for the experienced physician.

- First-degree (superficial) burns affect the skin's outer layer (epidermis). Characteristics include redness, mild swelling, tenderness, and pain. The outer edges of deeper burns are first-degree burns.

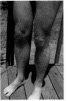

First-degree burn

- Second-degree (partial-thickness) burns extend through the entire outer layer and into the inner layer of skin. Blisters, swelling, weeping of fluids, and severe pain characterize these burns.

Second-degree burn blisters

- Third-degree (full-thickness) burns penetrate all the skin layers and into the underlying fat and muscle. The skin looks charred, leathery, or pearly gray. The skin does not blanch when pressed because the area is dead. No pain exists because the nerve endings have been damaged or destroyed. Any pain felt with this burn is caused by surrounding burns of lesser degrees.

B

4 Determine the size of the burn. A rough guide known as the "rule of nines" assigns a percentage value to each part of an adult's body. For small children and infants, the head accounts for 18 percent and each leg is 14 percent.

Rule of Nines is used to calculate the extent of a burn.

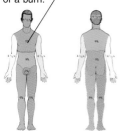

For small or scattered burns, use the "rule of the hand;" that is, one side of the victim's hand represents about one percent of his or her body surface.

5 After determining the information in steps 3 through 4, use the American Burn Association guidelines (see the accompanying table) to determine the burn's severity. Most burns are minor, occur at home, and can be managed outside of a medical setting.

Seek medical attention if any of these conditions exist:

- Burn is rated as moderate or severe using American Burn Association table
- Victim's age is under five or over sixty years
- Difficulty breathing
- Severe injuries exist
- Electric injury exists
- Face, hands, feet, or genitals burned
- Suspected child abuse
- Body surface area of
  —second-degree burn greater than 20 percent of the body surface
  —all third-degree burns

6 Care for a burn according to its severity (depth and size).

B

Burn Severity

Burn classification	Characteristics	
Minor burn	first-degree burn	
	second-degree burn	< 15% BSA adults
	second-degree burn	< 5% BSA in children/elderly persons
	third-degree burn	< 2% BSA
Moderate burn	second-degree burn	15%–25% BSA in adults
	second-degree burn	10%–20% BSA in children/elderly persons
	third-degree burn	< 10% BSA
Critical burn	second-degree burn	> 25% BSA in adults
	second-degree burn	> 20% BSA in children/elderly persons
	third-degree burn	> 10% BSA
		Burns of hands, face, eyes, feet, or perineum
		Most victims with inhalation injury, electrical injury, major trauma, or significant preexisting diseases

BSA = Body surface area
Source: Adapted with permission from the American Burn Association categorization.

B

Care of First-degree and Small Second-degree Burns

1 If the burned body surface area is less than 20 percent, place the burned area in cold water or apply a wet, cold cloth. Apply cold treatment until the part is pain free both in and out of the water (10 to 45 minutes). Cold treatment also stops the burn's progression into deeper tissue.

If cold water is unavailable, you can use any cold liquid clean enough to drink to reduce the burned skin's temperature.

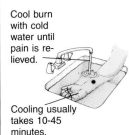

Cool burn with cold water until pain is relieved.

Cooling usually takes 10-45 minutes.

2 Relieve pain and inflammation by giving the victim aspirin or ibuprofen. Acetaminophen relieves pain but not inflammation.

After-care of minor (first-degree and small second-degree) burns when medical care is not needed

First-degree Burns

1 An anti-inflammatory drug (i.e., aspirin or ibuprofen) can reduce pain and swelling.

2 Aloe vera gel (100 percent) soothes and keeps the skin moist.

3 A dressing is not usually needed.

Second-degree Burns

1 Wash the burn very gently with lukewarm water and mild soap (i.e., baby shampoo, mild dish soap). Do not intentionally break blisters.

2 Apply a thin layer of antibiotic ointment (i.e., Bacitracin).

3 Wrap a nonsticking sterile dressing keeping it in place with roller gauze bandage. Covering burns reduces pain and fluid loss.

4   Re-dress once or twice daily by removing old dressings (you may have to soak them off with clean, lukewarm water), rewashing, and reapplying Bacitracin ointment, sterile non-stick dressing, and roller gauze bandage.

5   Elevate burned extremities to reduce swelling.

6   An anti-inflammatory drug (i.e., aspirin or ibuprofen) can relieve pain and swelling.

Care of Third-degree and Large Second-degree Burns

1   Cover the burn with a dry, nonsticking, sterile dressing or clean, dry cloth or sheet.

2   Treat for shock by elevating the legs and keeping the victim warm with a clean sheet or blanket. Raise burned arms or legs.

3   Seek medical attention.

CHEST INJURIES

Chest injuries are of two types: lung injuries and chest wall injuries (ribs).

Check the ABCHs. Keep a conscious chest injured victim sitting up or with the head and shoulders elevated. Another option is to place the victim with the injured side down. This protects the uninjured side from blood inside the chest cavity and allows the good lung to expand.

Seek medical attention for all chest injuries.

Broken Rib

Pain when breathing, coughing, or moving can indicate a broken rib.

WHAT TO DO

1 Stabilize the ribs by having the victim hold a pillow or similar soft object, or lightly wrap an elastic bandage to hold it against the injured area.

2 Tell the victim to take deep breaths and to cough several times each hour to prevent pneumonia.

Flail Chest

Several ribs next to each other broken in two or more places is called a flail chest. The victim's chest wall may move in the opposite direction to the rest of the chest wall during breathing (known as "paradoxical breathing").

Stabilize the chest by one of several methods:

- Apply hand pressure. This is useful for a short time.
- Place the victim on the injured side with a blanket or clothing underneath.

Penetrating Wound

Stabilize the object in place with bulky dressings. DO NOT try to remove a penetrating object; this may cause bleeding and allow air into the chest cavity.

Stabilize penetrating object with bulky padding.

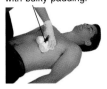
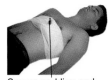

Secure padding and object.

Sucking Chest Wound

This happens when a chest wound allows air to pass into and out of the chest with each breath.

WHAT TO DO

1 Have the victim take a breath and let it out; then seal the wound with anything available to stop air from entering the chest cavity. Plastic wrap or bag works well. Tape the plastic in place with one corner untaped. This cre- ates a flutter valve that prevents air from being trapped in the chest cavity.

2 If the victim has trouble breathing or seems to be getting worse, remove the plastic cover to let air escape, then reapply.

CHEST PAIN

Many causes of chest pain exist:

- Muscle or rib pain from exercise or injury. The victim can reproduce the pain by move- ment, and often the painful area is tender when pushed on. Rest and aspirin or ibupro- fen provide relief.
- Respiratory infection (i.e., pneumonia, bron- chitis, or pleuritis) or lung injury is usually made worse by coughing and deep breathing. Fever and colored sputum may be present. Seek medical attention.
- Indigestion usually accompanied by burping, belching, heartburn, nausea, and a sour taste in the mouth. This type of pain is relieved by antacids.
- Heart attack. See page 21 for details.
- Angina pectoris. This happens when the heart muscle does not get as much blood (which means a lack of oxygen) as it needs. The pain is brought on by physical exertion, exposure to cold, emotional stress, or ingestion of food. It seldom lasts longer than 10 minutes and al- most always is relieved by nitroglycerin. A heart attack's chest pain is as likely to happen

at rest as during activity. The pain lasts longer than 10 minutes and is not relieved by nitroglycerin.

WHAT TO DO

1 Determine if the victim has physician-prescribed medicine for angina and, if the victim is conscious, help him or her take it. (Nitroglycerin comes as tablets, a spray for under the tongue, or in ointment that is placed on the skin.)

2 If the pain stops within 10 minutes, suspect angina. If the pain continues for more than 10 minutes, suspect a heart attack (see page 21).

DENTAL/MOUTH INJURIES

Seek a dentist for all dental emergencies.

Bitten Lip or Tongue

WHAT TO DO

1 Apply direct pressure to the bleeding area with sterile gauze or clean cloth.

2 If swelling is present, apply an ice pack or have the victim suck on an ice cube.

Knocked-Out Tooth

A knocked-out tooth may be successfully reimplanted in its socket. Save the tooth for a dentist to look at. Place a sterile gauze pad into tooth socket to control bleeding.

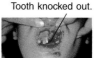

Tooth knocked out.

WHAT TO DO

1 Find and save the tooth. Handle it by the crown only. DO NOT scrub the tooth or remove any attached tissue fragments.

2 Place the tooth in a cup of milk or a commercial tooth-preserving solution. DO NOT put the tooth in mouthwash, alcohol, or water.

3 DO NOT remove a partially extracted tooth. Push it back into place.

4 Seek a dentist to stabilize the loose tooth or to replace the knocked-out tooth.

5 If you are in a remote area with no dentist nearby, replant a knocked-out tooth by:

- Handling it by the crown only, not the root
- Gently rinsing it with cool water to clean away dirt (do not scrub the tooth)
- Replacing it into the socket, using adjacent teeth as a guide
- Pushing the tooth so the top is even with the adjacent teeth: biting down gently on gauze is helpful

Broken Tooth

WHAT TO DO

1 Gently clean dirt and blood from the injured area with a sterile gauze pad or clean cloth and warm water.

2 Cover tooth with a sterile gauze.

Broken teeth

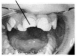

3 Apply an ice pack on the face in the area of the injured tooth to decrease swelling.

4 If a jaw fracture is suspected, stabilize the jaw by tying a bandage over and under the chin and over the top of the head.

D

Toothache

WHAT TO DO

1 Rinse the mouth with warm water to clean it out.

2 Use dental floss to remove any food that might be trapped between the teeth.

3 If a cavity is suspected, insert a small cotton ball soaked in oil of cloves (eugenol). Aspirin, acetamino-phen, or ibuprofen may be given for the pain. DO NOT place aspirin on the aching tooth or gum tissues. A serious acid burn can result.

4 Apply an ice pack on the face in the area of the aching tooth.

DIABETIC EMERGENCIES

D

Diabetes is a condition in which insulin, a hormone that helps the body use the energy in food, is either lacking or ineffective.

The body is continuously balancing sugar and insulin. Too much insulin and not enough sugar equals insulin shock or low blood sugar. Too much sugar and not enough insulin equals diabetic coma or high blood sugar.

The American Diabetes Association lists the following as signs and symptoms of diabetic emergencies and first aid.

WHAT TO LOOK FOR

Low Blood Sugar (Insulin Reaction or Hypoglycemia)

An insulin reaction happens when a person with diabetes takes too much insulin or eats too little food after taking insulin or other diabetes medications. Quick action is needed for this condition. See page 27 for details.

High Blood Sugar (Diabetic Coma, Hyperglycemia, or Acidosis)

- Gradual onset
- Drowsiness
- Extreme thirst
- Very frequent urination
- Flushed skin
- Vomiting
- Fruity or winelike breath odor
- Heavy breathing
- Eventual unconsciousness

WHAT TO DO

1 If you are uncertain whether high or low blood sugar exists, give food or drink containing sugar.

2 Give fluids.

3 If the victim does not get better in 15 minutes, the victim needs medical attention. Take the victim to the hospital.

DISLOCATION

A dislocation occurs when a joint (i.e., shoulder, finger) comes apart and stays apart with the bone ends no longer in contact. Symptoms of dislocation are similar to those of a broken bone: deformity, severe pain, swelling, and inability to move the injured joint.

WHAT TO DO

1 Check the **CSM** (circulation, sensation, movement).

2 Stabilize the part as if it were broken (see page 39).

3 DO NOT move the joint—nerves and blood vessels could be damaged. If there is no pulse, straighten the joint slightly.

4 Seek medical attention.

ELECTROCUTION

The major damage occurs inside the body, while the burn may appear small and is only seen on the outside.

WHAT TO DO

1 Make sure the area is safe. Either unplug, disconnect, or turn off the power. If this is impossible, call the power company or the EMS for help.

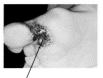

Electrical burn (toe)

2 Check and recheck the ABCs (see page 14).

3 Check for a spine injury (see page 35).

4 Treat for shock (see page 79).

5 Treat entry and exit burns (see page 42).

6 Seek medical attention immediately.

E

EYE INJURIES

All eye injuries are serious because they can lead to loss of sight or infection.

Seek immediate medical attention for all eye injuries.

Penetrating Injuries

Most penetrating injuries will be obvious. Suspect penetration any time you see a lid laceration or cut.

WHAT TO DO

1 DO NOT remove an object stuck in the eye.

2 Protect the injured eye with padding around the

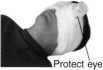

Protect eye and object with paper cup.

object. Place a paper cup or cardboard folded into a cone, to protect the eye and prevent the object from being driven deeper into the eye.

3 Cover the undamaged eye with a patch to stop movement of the damaged eye.

Blows to the Eye

E

WHAT TO DO

1 Apply a cold pack immediately for about 15 minutes to reduce pain and swelling.

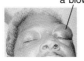

Swelling from a blow.

2 Seek medical attention immediately in cases of pain, reduced vision, or discoloration ("black eye").

Cuts of the Eye and Lid

WHAT TO DO

1 Bandage both eyes lightly. DO NOT apply hard pressure

to the injured eye (vision may be affected).

Chemical Burns

Alkalis cause greater damage than acids because they penetrate deeper and continue to burn longer. Common alkalis are drain cleaners, cleaning agents, ammonia, cement, plaster, and caustic soda. Common acids are hydrochloric acid, nitric acid, sulfuric (battery) acid, and acetic acid.

Damage can happen within 1 to 5 minutes, so speed in removing the chemical is vital.

See page 25 for WHAT TO DO.

Eye Avulsion

A blow to the eye can knock (avulse) it out of its socket.

WHAT TO DO

1 Cover the eye loosely with a sterile dressing that has been moistened with clean water. DO NOT try to push the eye back into the socket.

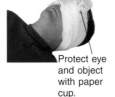
Protect eye and object with paper cup.

2 Protect the injured eye with a paper cup, cardboard folded into a cone, or doughnut-shaped pad made from a roller gauze bandage or a cravat bandage.

3 Cover the undamaged eye with a patch to stop movement of the damaged eye.

Foreign Objects

Foreign objects in an eye are the most frequent eye injury. They can be very painful.

WHAT TO DO

1 DO NOT allow the victim to rub the eye. DO NOT try to remove an embedded foreign object.

2 Lift the upper lid over the lower lid, allowing the lashes to brush the object off the inside of the upper lid. Blink a few times and let the eye move the object out. If the object remains, keep the eye closed.

3 Try flushing the object out by rinsing the eye gently with warm water. Hold the eyelid open and tell the victim to move the eye as it is rinsed.

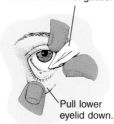

Remove with wet gauze.

Pull lower eyelid down.

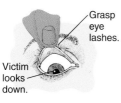

Grasp eye lashes.

Victim looks down.

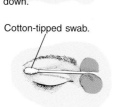

Cotton-tipped swab.

Roll eyelid over swab. Remove with wet gauze.

4 Examine the lower lid by pulling it down gently. Have the victim look up. If the object is seen, remove it with a moistened sterile gauze or clean cloth.

5 Examine the upper lid by grasping the lashes of the upper lid, placing a match stick or cotton-tipped swab across the upper lid, and rolling the lid upward over the stick or swab. Have the victim look down. If the object is seen, remove it with a moistened sterile gauze or clean cloth.

Light Burns

These injuries result from looking at ultraviolet light (i.e., sunlight, arc welding, bright snow, tanning lamps). Severe pain develops 1 to 6 hours after exposure.

WHAT TO DO

1 Cover both eyes with cold, wet packs.

2 An analgesic for pain may be needed. DO NOT allow the victim to rub the eye.

Contact Lenses

An eye-injured victim wearing contact lenses must have them removed as soon as possible. Usually the victim can effectively remove the lenses.

FAINTING

Fainting (brief loss of consciousness) can happen suddenly or the victim may feel it coming (i.e., dizziness, nausea, weakness).

WHAT TO DO

If a person appears about to faint:

1 Prevent the person from falling.

2 Have the person lie down and raise the legs 8 to 12 inches.

3 Loosen tight clothing, especially from around the neck.

4 Place cool, wet cloth on forehead.

If a person has fainted:

1 Check the ABCHs.

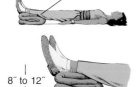

Keep legs straight.

8″ to 12″

2 Lay the victim down and raise the legs 8 to 12 inches unless a head injury due to the fall is suspected.

3 Loosen tight clothing, especially from around the neck.

4 If the victim fell, check for injuries.

5 Place a cool, wet cloth on forehead. DO

NOT splash or pour water on the victim's face.

6 DO NOT try to revive victim by using smelling salts or ammonia inhalants, by slapping the victim's face, or by giving something to drink.

7 Seek medical attention if the victim does not fully recover within 5 minutes or complains of being ill.

FINGER/TOE INJURIES

Broken/Dislocated

Use the "tapping" test by having the victim hold the fingers or toes in full extension on a solid surface (i.e., table top). Firmly tap the end of the victim's finger or toe toward the victim's hand or foot, transmitting the force down the shaft of the finger's or toe's bones. If this tapping produces additional pain, suspect a broken bone.

Tap the end of a victim's finger toward hand.

WHAT TO DO

1 Stabilize the finger/toe by either:

- Using tape to attach it to an adjacent finger/toe, or
- Placing the hand and fingers into what is called the "position of function" (finger flexed as it would be when comfortably holding a baseball). A wad of bulky dressings or cloths is then placed in the hand and secured with a roller bandage on a board or folded newspapers.

2 Seek medical attention.

Nail Avulsion

If nail is partly torn or loose, secure the damaged nail in place with an adhesive bandage.
If part or all of the nail has been completely torn away, apply antibiotic ointment and secure with an adhesive bandage over the nail. DO NOT trim away the loose nail.

Splinters

If a splinter passes under a nail and breaks off flush, remove the embedded part by grasping its end with tweezers after cutting a V-shaped notch in the nail to gain access to the splinter.
If a splinter is in the skin, tease it out with a sterile needle until the end can be grasped with tweezers or fingers.

Bleeding Under a Finger or Toe Nail

After a direct blow to a nail, blood can collect under the nail, resulting in severe pain.

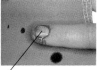

Relieve pain by releasing blood under a nail.

F

WHAT TO DO

1 Place the finger in cold water or apply an ice pack while keeping the hand raised.

2 Relieve pain caused by blood under the nail by either:

• Drilling through the nail with a rotary action with the sharp point of a knife (this can be painful), or

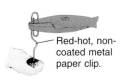

Red-hot, non-coated metal paper clip.

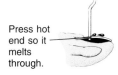

Press hot end so it melts through.

• Straightening the end of a metal (noncoated) wire paper clip or using the end (with the hole) of a sewing needle. Hold the paper clip or needle with pliers and heat it until red hot with a match or cigarette lighter. Press the glowing end of the paper clip or needle so it melts through the nail. Very little pressure is needed. The nail has no nerves, so it is painless.

3 Apply a dressing to absorb the draining blood and to protect the injured nail.

Ring Removal

Sometimes a finger is too swollen to remove a ring and circulation can be cut off if the ring is left on too long. If the ring is not removed, gangrene could develop within 4 or 5 hours. Try one or more of these methods:

• Lubricate the finger with grease, oil, butter, petroleum jelly, or some other slippery substance, then try to remove the ring, or
• Place the finger in cold water or apply an ice pack for several minutes to reduce the swelling, or
• Massage the finger from the tip to the hand to move the swelling; lubricate the finger again and try removing the ring, or
• If still unsuccessful, try one or more of these:

1 Slip the end of a string under the ring with a matchstick or toothpick. Smoothly wind string around the finger, starting about an inch from the ring's edge and going toward the ring with one strand touching the next. Continue winding smoothly and tightly right up to the edge of the ring. This will push the swelling toward the hand. Slowly unwind the string on the hand side of the ring. You should then be able to twist the ring gently off the finger over the string.

2 Cut the narrowest part of the ring with a ring saw, jeweler's saw, ring cutter, triangular file or fine hacksaw blade. Protect the exposed portions of the finger.

3 Inflate an ordinary balloon (preferably a slender, tube-shaped one) about three-fourths full. Tie the end. Push the victim's swollen finger into the end of the balloon so that the balloon rolls back evenly around the finger. In about 15 minutes, the finger should return to its normal size and the ring can be removed.

FROSTBITE

F

Frostbite, the freezing of skin and underlying tissues, happens only in below-freezing temperatures. The skin feels cold and firm and looks white or bluish. The victim has no feeling and will say the part feels numb.

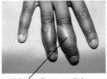

Frostbitten fingers 6 hours after rewarming in 108° F water.

A less serious condition is *frostnip*. The skin becomes white or pale and remains pliable. First aid for frostnip consists of

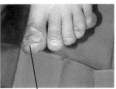

Third degree frostbite

gently warming the affected area with bare hands or by blowing warm air on the area. After rewarming, the area may be red, tender, and slightly swollen.

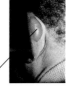

Frostbitten ear 8 hours old.

WHAT TO DO

1 Get the victim out of the cold and to a warm place. Remove any constrictive clothing or items.

2 Seek medical attention immediately.

If the victim is in a remote or wilderness area (more than 2 hours from medical attention), use the wet, rapid rewarming method:

1 Place the frostbitten part in warm water (102° to 106°). Rewarming usually takes 20 to 40 minutes or until the tissue is soft. Help control the severe pain during rewarming by giving aspirin or ibuprofen. DO NOT rub or massage or use snow or ice on the part. DO NOT allow the victim to drink alcoholic beverages or smoke.

2 After thawing:

• Treat victim as a "stretcher" case because feet will be impossible to use once rewarmed.

• Protect victim from objects such as clothing and bedding.

• Place dry, sterile gauze between toes and fingers.

• Slightly elevate the affected part to reduce pain and swelling.

• Give aspirin or ibuprofen to limit pain and swelling.

• Prevent refreezing.

HEAD INJURIES

Scalp Wounds

Scalp wounds bleed profusely because of the rich blood supply. Suspect a spinal injury to the neck.

WHAT TO DO

1 Control bleeding by applying direct pressure (see page 18).

2 If a skull fracture is suspected, apply pressure around the edges of the wound (use a doughnut-shaped pad) and over a broad area rather than at its center. DO NOT clean the wound or irrigate it.

3 Slightly raise head and shoulders to help control bleeding

4 DO NOT remove a penetrating object; instead, stabilize it in place with bulky dressings.

Skull Fracture

A skull fracture is a break or crack in the bony casing surrounding the brain.

WHAT TO LOOK FOR

Skull fractures are extremely difficult to detect except by x-ray examination unless the skull deformity is severe. Some signs are:

- Pain at the point of injury
- Deformity of the skull and pain
- Bleeding or leakage of a clear, pink, watery fluid from the ears and/or nose
- Discoloration around the eyes or behind an ear that appears several hours after the injury
- A scalp wound exposing skull or brain tissue
- Penetrating wound (i.e., bullet)

WHAT TO DO

1 Check the ABCHs

2 Cover wounds with a sterile dressing

3 Stabilize neck against movement

4 Slightly raise head and shoulders to help control bleeding

5 Apply pressure around wound edges (use doughnut-shaped pad), not directly on the wound.

6   DO NOT stop the flow of blood or clear fluid from an ear or nose.

7   DO NOT remove a penetrating object from the head. Stabilize it in place with bulky dressings.

8   DO NOT clean or irrigate an open skull fracture.

Brain Injuries

When the head is struck with sufficient force, the brain is "bounced around" within the skull. The brain, like other body tissue, swells when injured. Unlike other tissue, the brain is confined within the rigid skull, where little additional space is available to accommodate swelling. Therefore, a brain injury can increase intracranial pressure, which can reduce the blood supply to the brain. Brain injuries are frequently classified as:

- *Concussion:* A temporary loss of brain function, usually without permanent damage. No bleeding in the brain occurs.
- *Contusion:* Brain tissue is bruised.
- *Hematoma:* Localized collection of blood as a result of a broken blood vessel. This is the most serious of the brain injuries.

WHAT TO LOOK FOR

Increased pressure on the brain will show:

- Memory loss
- Vomiting and nausea
- Headache, vision disturbance, loss of balance
- Unequal pupils
- Weakness or paralysis
- Seizures
- Blood or clear fluid (cerebrospinal fluid) leakage from ears or nose
- Combativeness—the victim strikes out ran-

domly and with surprising strength at the nearest person
- Unconsciousness

The signs and symptoms of brain injury can go unnoticed for the first 6 to 18 hours. As the swelling expands, the signs and symptoms become more evident.

Ask a conscious victim what day it is, where he or she is, and personal questions such as birthday and home address. If the victim cannot answer these questions, there may be a significant problem. Another useful test is to give a list of five or six numbers and ask the victim to repeat them in the same order. Failing these short-term memory tests indicates a concussion.

WHAT TO DO

1 Seek medical attention immediately for all brain-injured victims

2 Suspect a spinal injury. Stabilize the victim's head and neck as you found them either by:

Gently squeeze head between forearms.

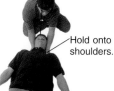
Hold onto shoulders.

- Using your hands and forearms along both sides of the head, or

- Placing soft but rigid materials alongside the head and neck.

3 Check the ABCHs.

4 Control scalp bleeding (see page 62).

5 Brain-injured victims tend to vomit. Rolling the victim as a unit onto his or her left side while stabilizing the neck against movement will help prevent vomiting and also drain vomit while keeping the airway open.

6 If no spinal injury is suspected, slightly

H

raise head and shoulders to help control bleeding and to prevent increased pressure within the brain.

7 DO NOT stop the flow of blood or clear fluid from an ear or nose.

8 DO NOT give the victim anything to eat or drink.

HEAT ILLNESSES

Heat Index

Relative Humidity	Air Temperature										
	70	75	80	85	90	95	100	105	110	115	120
	Apparent Temperature*										
0%	64	69	73	78	83	87	91	95	99	103	107
10%	65	70	75	80	85	90	95	100	105	111	116
20%	66	72	77	82	87	93	99	105	112	120	130
30%	67	73	78	84	90	96	104	113	123	135	148
40%	68	74	79	86	93	101	110	123	137	151	
50%	69	75	81	88	96	107	120	135	150		
60%	70	76	82	90	100	114	132	149			
70%	70	77	85	93	106	124	144				
80%	71	78	86	97	113	136					
90%	71	79	88	102	122						
100%	72	80	91	108							

Above 130°F = heat stroke imminent
105°–130° = heat exhaustion and heat cramps likely and heat stroke with long exposure and activity
90°–105° = heat exhaustion and heat cramps with long exposure and activity
80°–90° = fatigue during exposure and activity

*Degrees Fahrenheit
Source: National Weather Service

Heat Stroke

Heat stroke is a life-threatening emergency! Untreated victims always die. If death does not result, the high body temperature will damage tissues and organs throughout the body. Every minute of delay increases the likelihood of serious complications or death. (See page 23 for WHAT TO DO.)

Heat Exhaustion

Heat exhaustion results from sweating a lot and not drinking enough to replace lost body salt and water after a prolonged time in a hot environment.

WHAT TO LOOK FOR

You can tell the difference between heat exhaustion and heat stroke:

1. *Temperature.* Heat exhaustion is normal; heat stroke usually has a high temperature.
2. *Mental status.* Heat exhaustion is normal; heat stroke has altered or changed mental status.

WHAT TO DO

1 Move the victim to a cool place and remove any excess clothing.

2 Raise the victim's legs 8 to 12 inches (keep legs straight).

3 Give the victim cold water mixed with ¼ to 1 level teaspoon of salt in a quart of water or a commercial electrolyte drink. If no salted fluids are available, give cold water. DO NOT give salt tablets.

4 Sponge with cool water and fan victim.

5 If no improvement is seen within 30 minutes, seek medical attention.

Heat Cramps

Heat cramps are sudden, painful muscle spasms affecting legs (usually calf muscles) or abdominal muscles. The exact cause of heat cramps (and other similar cramps, such as exercise-induced cramps, nocturnal cramps, writer's cramps) is unknown. Heat cramps usually happen after several hours of hard physical activity in individuals who have lost a lot of sweat or have drunk a lot of unsalted fluid.

WHAT TO DO

1 Move victim to a cool place.

2 Stretch the cramping muscle. DO NOT massage the cramping muscle.

3 Give victim cold water mixed with 1/4 to 1 level teaspoon of salt in a quart of water or a commercial electrolyte drink. If no salted fluids are available, give cold water. DO NOT give salt tablets.

4 Try the accupressure method of pinching the upper lip for relief.

Other Heat Illnesses

- *Prickly heat* (heat rash) is an itchy rash that develops on skin moist from sweating. Treat by drying and cooling the skin.
- *Heat swelling* is mild swelling of the hands, feet, or ankles. It is common in people not acclimatized to a hot environment and is usually self-correcting. Wearing support stockings and elevating the legs may reduce the swelling.
- *Heat syncope* is fainting while standing in a hot environment. Use the same method of treatment as for fainting. However, fainting during or after work in the heat or after several days of heat exposure could indicate heat exhaustion or heat stroke.

HYPERVENTILATION

Hyperventilation is breathing faster and more deeply than normal because of anxiety or emotional stress.

WHAT TO LOOK FOR

- Fast, heavy breathing
- Dizziness
- Numbness and tingling in the hands and around the mouth and lips
- Chest pain
- Sweating

WHAT TO DO

1 Have victim lie down in a quiet place for 15 to 30 minutes.

2 Coach the victim to breathe slowly. DO NOT have him or her breathe into a paper bag because a more serious medical condition may be affected.

3 Reassure and calm the victim.

4 If the victim faints, treat for fainting (see page 57).

HYPOTHERMIA

Hypothermia is a life-threatening emergency! It can develop at temperatures above freezing as well as below, indoors or outdoors. The victim may also suffer frostbite.

WHAT TO LOOK FOR

- Mild (body temperature above 90° F): shivering, slurred speech, memory lapses, and fumbling hands. Victims frequently stumble and stagger. They are usually conscious and can talk. While many people suffer cold hands and feet, victims of mild hypothermia experience cold abdomens and backs.
- Severe (body temperature below 90° F): Shivering has stopped. Muscles may be stiff and rigid, similar to rigor mortis. The victim's skin is ice cold and has a blue appearance. Pulse and breathing slow down; pupils dilate. The victim appears to be dead.

How Cold Is It?

In addition to coldness, two other factors account for body heat loss: moisture and wind. Moisture—whether from rain, snow, or perspiration—speeds the conduction of heat away from the body.

Wind causes sizable amounts of body heat loss. If the thermometer reads 20°F and the wind speed is 20 mph, the exposure is comparable to −10°F. This is called the wind-chill factor. A rough measure of wind speed is: If you feel the wind on your face, the speed is about 10 mph; if small branches move or dust or snow is raised, 20 mph; if large branches are moving, 30 mph; and if a whole tree bends, about 40 mph.

Determine the wind-chill factor by:
1. Estimating the wind speed by checking for the signs described above.
2. Looking at a thermometer reading (in Fahrenheit degrees) outdoors.
3. Determining the wind-chill factor by matching the estimated wind speed with the actual thermometer reading in the "Wind-Chill Factor" table.

H

Wind Chill Factor	Actual Thermometer Reading (°F)											
Estimated Wind Speed (in MPH)	Equivalent Temperature (°F)											
	50	40	30	20	10	0	−10	−20	−30	−40	−50	−60
calm	50	40	30	20	10	0	−10	−20	−30	−40	−50	−60
5	48	37	27	16	6	−5	−15	−26	−36	−47	−57	−68
10	40	28	16	4	−9	−24	−33	−46	−58	−70	−83	−95
15	36	22	9	−5	−18	−32	−45	−58	−72	−85	−99	−112
20	32	18	4	−10	−25	−39	−53	−67	−82	−96	−110	−124
25	30	16	0	−15	−29	−44	−59	−74	−88	−104	−118	−133
30	25	13	−2	−18	−33	−48	−63	−79	−94	−109	−125	−140
35	27	11	−4	−20	−35	−51	−67	−82	−98	−113	−129	−145
40	26	10	−6	−21	−37	−53	−69	−85	−100	−116	−132	−148
(Wind speeds greater than 40 mph have little additional effect.)	Little danger (for properly clothed person). Maximum danger of false sense of security.				Increasing danger. (Flesh may freeze within 1 minute.)				Great danger. (Flesh may freeze within 30 seconds.)			

WHAT TO DO

1 Keep victim in horizontal (flat) position and handle the victim very gently.

2 Seek medical attention immediately.

3 *For all hypothermic victims,* stop further heat loss by

- Getting the victim out of the cold
- Having a source of heat (i.e., stove, fire) and adding heat to the victim.

This is not "re-warming" the victim.

- Adding insulation beneath and around the victim. Cover the victim's head because 50 percent of the body's heat loss is through the head.
- Replacing wet clothing with dry clothing

For a remote or wilderness situation

Mild Hypothermia

Raise the core body temperature by using one of these methods:

- Warm water immersion method: This method requires a lot of hot water (102° to 106° F) and a bathtub. Leave victim's arms and legs out of the warm water and elevated.
- Hot packs method: This is useful when combined with the sleeping bag method below. Place hot packs against the body's areas of high heat loss (i.e., neck, armpits, and groin). Do not burn victim.
- Sleeping bag method: Have a rescuer lie trunk to trunk with the victim in a sleeping bag.

Severe or Profound hypothermia

- Check victim's ABCs (airway, breathing, circulation). Take 30 to 45 seconds to check the pulse.

H

- Provide as much heat as possible. Adding heat and providing insulation does not mean you are "rewarming" the victim.
- Transport the victim by helicopter. Rewarming at a remote scene is difficult and rarely effective.

MUSCLE INJURIES

Muscle strain, also known as a muscle pull, occurs when a muscle is stretched beyond its normal range of motion, resulting in a muscle tearing. Use the **RICE** procedures (see page 108).

Muscle contusions (bruise) result from a blow to a muscle. Use the **RICE** procedures (see page 108).

Muscle cramps are uncontrolled muscle spasms and contractions that cause severe pain and loss of movement.

M

WHAT TO DO

1 Have the victim gently stretch the affected muscle. DO NOT massage or rub the affected muscle.

2 Pinch the upper lip (an accupressure technique) to reduce cramping of the calf muscle.

3 Give mildly salted water (1/4 to 1 level teaspoon in 1 quart of water) or a commercial sports drink . DO NOT give salt tablets.

NOSE INJURIES

Nosebleeds

WHAT TO DO

1 Keep the victim in a sitting position with the head bent slightly forward so that blood will not run down the back of the throat.

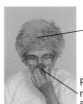

Keep head slightly bent forward.

Pinch both nostrils for 5 minutes.

2 Pinch both nostrils with steady pressure for 5 minutes. The victim can do the pinching.

3 If bleeding continues, have the victim gently blow the nose to remove any clots and excess blood, and to minimize sneezing. This allows new clots to form. Then press the nostrils again for 5 minutes.

4 If bleeding continues, seek medical attention.

If the victim is unconscious, place him or her on the side to prevent inhalation of blood and use the procedures listed above.

Objects in Nose

Foreign objects in the nose are a problem mainly for small children, who seem to gain some satisfaction from putting peanuts, beans, raisins, and similar objects into their nostrils. Determine which nostril is affected. Try one or all of these:

1 Induce sneezing by having the victim sniff pepper or by tickling the opposite nostril.

2 Have the victim blow her or his nose gently as the opposite nostril is pressed.

3 If the object is visible, use tweezers to pull it out. DO NOT probe or push an object deeper.

4 Seek medical attention if the object cannot be removed.

Broken Nose

WHAT TO DO

1 Treat a nosebleed as described above.

2 Apply an ice pack to the nose for 15 minutes.

3 Seek medical at-

N

tention. If a spinal injury is suspected, stabilize the head and neck and call the EMS.

POISON, SWALLOWED/INGESTED

Swallowed poisons usually remain in the stomach only a short time. Most absorption takes place after the poison passes into the small intestine. A poison is more dangerous in the intestines than in the stomach.

WHAT TO LOOK FOR

- Abdominal pain and cramping
- Nausea; vomiting
- Diarrhea
- Burns, odor, stains around and in mouth
- Drowsiness or unconsciousness
- Poison containers nearby

WHAT TO DO

1 Determine, if possible, this critical information:

- Who? Age and size of the victim.
- What was swallowed?
- How much was swallowed (a taste, half a bottle, etc.)?
- When was it swallowed?

If a corrosive or caustic (i.e., acid or alkali) was swallowed, immediately dilute with water or milk. DO NOT give water or milk to dilute other types of poisons unless instructed by a poison control center.

If the victim is unconscious, check the ABCs. Call the EMS.

2 Call a poison control center immediately. By following their advice, 70 percent of all poisonings can be handled outside of a medical facility.

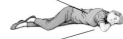

Place on left side.

Position for poisoned victim.

3 Keep all poisoned victims on the left side to delay stomach emptying into the small intestine, where a poison is absorbed faster. The side position also protects the lungs if vomiting begins.

4 DO NOT induce vomiting unless a poison control center or physician advises it. If advised, use syrup of ipecac with one to two glasses of water. DO NOT use salt water, raw eggs, mustard water, dishwashing liquid, or tickling the back of the throat to cause vomiting. If advised and available, give activated charcoal.

5 DO NOT follow a container label's first aid recommendations without getting confirmation from a poison control center.

6 Take any poison container, remaining portions of the substance swallowed, and vomit to the hospital with the victim.

P

POISON IVY, OAK, AND SUMAC

Poison ivy, oak, and sumac plants cause an allergic reaction (skin rash) in 50 percent of all adults. Although half will react, only 15 to 25 percent will have incapacitating swelling and blistering eruptions.

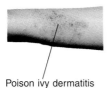

Poison ivy dermatitis

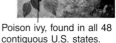

Poison ivy, found in all 48 contiguous U.S. states.

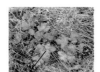

Poison oak

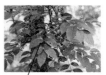

Poison sumac

Allergic people may come in contact with the oily resin (urushiol) of these plants from direct contact with the plant, their clothes or shoes, from pet fur, or from smoke of burning plants. No one can develop the dermatitis by touching the fluid from blisters, since that fluid does not contain the plant's oily resin.

WHAT TO LOOK FOR

- Mild: itching
- Mild to moderate: itching and redness
- Moderate: itching, redness, and swelling
- Severe: itching, redness, swelling, and blisters

Severity is important, but so is the amount of skin affected. The greater the amount of skin affected, the greater the need for medical attention.

WHAT TO DO

1 Those who know that they have contacted a poisonous plant should take immediate action (within 5 minutes). Most victims do not know about their contact until several hours or days later, when the itching and rash begin. Use soap and water promptly to clean the skin of the oily resin, or apply rubbing alcohol liberally (not in swab-type dabs). Other solvents can be used (i.e., paint thinner or gasoline), but they are hard on the skin. Rinse with water to remove the solubilized material off the skin.

2 For the mild stage, apply any of the following:

- Wet compresses soaked with Burow's solution (aluminum acetate), applied for 20 to 30 minutes three or four times a day
- Calamine lotion or zinc oxide
- Lukewarm bathwater sprinkled with one to two cups of Aveeno (colloidal oatmeal). Colloidal oatmeal makes a tub very slick, so warn the victim about its being slippery.
- Baking soda paste. Add one teaspoon of water to three teaspoons of baking soda, mix, and apply.

3 For the mild to moderate stage:

- Care for the skin as you would for the mild stage.
- Apply corticosteroid ointment as prescribed by a physician. Nonprescription hydrocortisone creams, ointments, and sprays are not effective.
- For itching, immerse the area or run hot water over it. The water should be hot enough to redden the skin, but not burn it. Heat releases histamine, the substance in the skin's cells that causes severe itching. As the histamine is released, the victim experiences intense itching. This depletes the cells of histamine, and the victim will then get up to 8 hours of relief from itching.

4 For the severe stage:

- Use a physician-prescribed oral corticosteroid (i.e., prednisone).
- Apply topical corticosteriod ointment or cream and cover with a transparent plastic wrap. Bind lightly with an elastic or self-adhering bandage.

P

SEIZURES

A seizure is the result of a sudden abnormal electrical stimulation of the brain. Seizures are not nearly as serious as they appear. You cannot stop a seizure. Several medical conditions can cause seizure, including:

- Epilepsy
- Heat stroke
- Poisoning or drug reaction
- Hypoglycemia (insulin shock)
- High fever in children
- Brain injury, tumor, or stroke
- Electric shock

Epileptic seizures may be convulsive or non-convulsive, depending on where in the brain the malfunction takes place and on how much of the total brain area is involved.

- Convulsive seizures are the ones most people think of when they hear the words "epilepsy" or "seizure." In this type of seizure, the person undergoes convulsions usually lasting from 2 to 5 minutes with muscle spasms and complete loss of consciousness.
- Nonconvulsive seizures may take the form of a blank stare lasting only a few seconds, an involuntary movement of an arm or leg, or a period of automatic movement in which awareness of one's surroundings is blurred or completely absent.

WHAT TO DO

The Epilepsy Foundation of American gives these procedures for convulsions, generalized tonic–clonic seizures, and grand mal seizures:

1 Cushion the victim's head with something soft (i.e., coat, blanket).

2 Loosen tight clothing around the victim's neck. DO NOT put anything between the victim's teeth during the seizure. DO NOT hold the victim down.

3 Turn the victim onto side.

4 Look for a medic alert tag (bracelet or necklace).

5 As seizure ends, offer your help. Most seizures in people with epilepsy are not medical emergencies. They end after a minute or two without harm and usually do not require medical attention. Avoid embarrassing victim by clearing away bystanders and covering person if bladder control failed. Reassure victim.

6 Call the EMS when:

- A seizure happens in someone who does not have epilepsy. It could be a sign of serious illness.
- A seizure lasts more than 5 minutes.
- There is no "epilepsy" or "seizure disorder" identification.
- Recovery is slow, there is a second seizure, or breathing is difficult afterward.
- Pregnancy or other medical condition is identified.
- Any signs of injury or illnesses are seen.

SHOCK

Shock is a life-threatening emergency! Prevention is easier than treating it after it happens. To understand shock, think of the circulatory system as having three parts: a working pump (the heart), a network of pipes (the blood vessels), and an adequate amount of fluid (the blood) pumped through the pipes. Damage to any of these parts can deprive tissues of blood and produce the condition known as shock.

WHAT TO LOOK FOR

- Pale or bluish and cool skin, nailbeds, and lips
- Moist and clammy skin
- Weakness
- Rapid pulse and breathing
- Nausea; vomiting
- Thirst
- Unconsciousness in severe cases

WHAT TO DO

Treat all injured victims for shock even if shock's signs and symptoms have not appeared in an injured victim.

1 Check the ABCHs. Treat life-threatening injuries and other injuries.

2 Lay the victim down on his or her back with the legs straight and raised 8 to 12 inches. DO NOT lift the foot of a

an unconscious victim on the side. If spinal injury is suspected, do not move victim.

3 Prevent loss of body heat by wrapping blankets, coats, etc., around the victim.

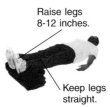

Raise legs
8-12 inches.

Keep legs
straight.

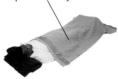

Use a blanket or coat
to prevent body heat

bed or stretcher. Those with breathing difficulties, head or chest injuries, and heart attacks should be placed in a half-sitting position. Place

4 DO NOT give the victim anything to eat or drink.

5 Seek medical attention.

SNAKEBITES

Only four snake species in the United States are poisonous: rattlesnake (accounts for about 65 percent of all venomous snakebites and nearly all snakebite deaths in the United States), copperhead, water moccasin, and coral snake. The first three are known as pit vipers because of the heat-sensitive "pit" between each eye and nostril.

Coral snake. America's most poisonous snake.

Rattlesnake

Copperhead snake

Cottonmouth water moccasin.

Copperhead bite two hours after bite.

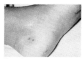
Rattlesnake bite. Note two fang marks.

S

Pit Viper Snakebite

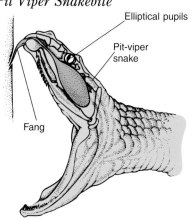
Elliptical pupils

Pit-viper snake

Fang

Location of Venomous Snakes

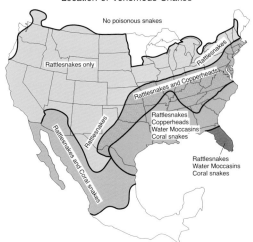

No poisonous snakes

Rattlesnakes only

Rattlesnakes and Copperheads

Rattlesnakes

Rattlesnakes
Copperheads
Water Moccasins
Coral snakes

Rattlesnakes and Coral snakes

Rattlesnakes
Water Moccasins
Coral snakes

S

WHAT TO LOOK FOR

- Severe, burning pain at the bite site
- Two small puncture wounds about 1/2 inch apart (some victims may have only one fang mark)
- Swelling (happens within 5 minutes and can involve an entire extremity)
- Discoloration and blood-filled blisters may develop within 6 to 10 hours
- In severe cases: nausea, vomiting, sweating, weakness
- No venom is injected in about 25 percent of all poisonous snakebites; only fang and tooth wounds (known as a "dry" bite) are present. These require only care of the bite wounds and possibly, a tetanus shot.

WHAT TO DO

1 Get the victim away from the snake. Snakes have been known to bite more than once. Be careful around a decapitated snake head because head reactions last for 20 minutes or more.

2   Keep the victim quiet. If possible, carry the victim or walk very slowly to help.

3   Gently wash the bitten area with soap and water.

4   If you are more than a few hours from a medical facility with antivenin, or if the snake was large and the skin is swelling rapidly, you should immediately apply suction with the Extractor (from Sawyer Products). This does not require the skin to be cut. Apply suction immediately and leave on for 30 minutes. This procedure is seldom needed because most bite victims are a short distance from a medical facility.

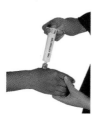

5   Seek medical attention immediately. This is the most important thing to do for the victim. Antivenin must be given within 4 hours of the bite. The same antivenin is used for all North American pit viper venom.

DO NOT use on snakebites:

- cold or ice—It does not inactivate the venom and poses a frostbite hazard.
- tourniquet—It increases the likelihood of losing the extremity.
- cut-and-suck method—There is a danger of damaging underlying structures (i.e., blood vessels, nerves).
- mouth suction—Your mouth is filled with bacteria, and can infect the snakebite victim's wound.
- electric shock—No medical studies support this method.

Coral Snakebite

The coral snake is America's most poisonous snake, but it rarely bites people. It has short fangs and tends to hang on and "chew" its venom into the victim rather than to strike and release like a pit viper.

WHAT TO DO

1 Keep the victim calm. DO NOT apply a constriction band or cut the victim's skin.

2 Gently clean bite site with soap and water.

3 Seek medical attention for antivenin.

Nonpoisonous Snakebite

Nonpoisonous snakes leave horseshoe-shaped toothmarks on victim's skin. When you are not positive about a snake, assume it was venomous. Some "nonpoisonous" North American snakes (i.e., hognose and garter snakes) have venom that can cause a painful local reaction but no whole-body symptoms.

WHAT TO DO

1 Gently clean bite site with soap and water.

2 Care for the bite as a minor wound.

3 Seek medical advice.

SPIDER BITES AND SCORPION STINGS

Few spiders have fangs long enough to bite humans. Exceptions include the black widow, brown recluse, and tarantula spiders.

Black Widow Spider

WHAT TO LOOK FOR

- The spider's bite may be felt as a sharp pinprick, although some victims are not even aware of the bite. Within 15 minutes a dull, numbing pain develops in the bitten area.

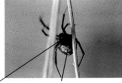

Black widow spider

Note red hourglass configuration on abdomen.

- Faint red bite marks appear.
- Muscle stiffness and cramps develop next, usually affecting the abdomen when the bite is in the lower part of the body or legs, and affecting the shoulders, back, or chest when the bite is on the upper body or arms.
- Headache, chills, fever, heavy sweating, dizziness, nausea, vomiting, and severe abdominal pain may occur.

Brown Recluse Spider

The brown recluse spider has a brown, possibly purplish, violin-shaped figure on its back.

Brown recluse spider

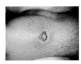

Brown recluse spider bite

WHAT TO LOOK FOR

- During the early stages, the affected area often takes on a bull's-eye appearance, with a central white area surrounded by a reddened area, ringed by a whitish or blue border. A blister at the bite site, along with redness and swelling, appears after several hours.

- Pain, which may remain mild but can become severe, develops within 2 to 8 hours at the bite site.
- Fever, weakness, vomiting, joint pain, and a rash may occur.

Tarantula

Tarantulas are large, hairy spiders. A tarantula's bite produces moderate pain.

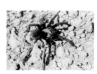
Tarantula

WHAT TO DO

For all spider bites:

1 If possible, catch the spider to confirm its identity. Even if the body is crushed, save it for identification.

2 Clean the bitten area with soap and water or rubbing alco-hol. DO NOT apply a constricting band.

3 Place an ice pack over the bite.

4 Check the ABCs.

5 Seek medical attention immediately.

Scorpion Stings

Scorpions look like little lobsters; they have lobsterlike pincers and a long upcurved "tail" with a poisonous stinger. A scorpion's sting causes immediate pain and burning around

Scorpion

the sting site, followed by numbness or tingling. Usually only children are affected severely, and their symptoms may include paralysis, spasms, or breathing difficulties.

WHAT TO DO

1 Check the ABCs.

2 Gently clean the bite site with soap and water or rubbing alcohol.

3 Apply an ice pack over the sting site.

4 Seek medical attention.

STINGS, INSECT

Stinging insects include the honeybee, bumble-bee, yellow jacket, hornet, wasp, and fire ant. For the severely allergic person, a single sting may be fatal within minutes.

WHAT TO LOOK FOR

The sooner symptoms develop after the sting, the more serious the reaction will be. Reactions generally occur within a few minutes to 1 hour after the sting.

- Usual reactions: momentary pain, redness around sting site, itching, heat
- Worrisome reactions: skin flush, hives, localized swelling of lips or tongue, "tickle" in throat, wheezing, abdominal cramps, diarrhea
- Life-threatening reactions: Bluish or grayish skin color, seizures, unconsciousness, inability to breathe due to swelling of vocal cords

One of the difficulties in dealing with stings is the lack of uniformity in victims' responses. One sting is not necessarily equivalent to another, even within the same species, because the amount of venom injected varies from sting to sting.

WHAT TO DO

1 Look at the sting site for a stinger embedded in the skin. Only the honeybee leaves its stinger embedded. If the stinger is still embedded, remove it by scraping with a long fingernail, credit card, scissor edge, or knife blade. Unless removed, the stinger will continue to inject poison for 2 or 3 minutes. DO NOT pull the stinger with tweezers or fingers because more venom may be squeezed into the victim from the venom sac.

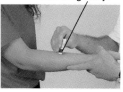
Scrape the honey bee sting away.

2   Wash the sting site with soap and water.

3   Apply an ice pack over the sting site to slow absorption of the venom and relieve pain.

4   Apply Secta Sooth Sting Relief Swab or Sting Eze to the sting site.

5   To relieve pain and itching further, give aspirin or acetaminophen. An antihistamine may prevent some local symptoms if given early, but it works too slowly to counteract a life-threatening allergic reaction.

6   Observe victims for at least 30 minutes for signs of an allergic reaction. For those having a severe allergic reaction, a dose of epinephrine is the only effective life-saving treatment. Ask the victim if he or she has a physician-prescribed emergency kit that includes a pre-filled syringe of epinephrine or a spring-loaded device that automatically triggers the injection of epinephrine by a quick thrust into the thigh or large muscle. Because epinephrine is short-acting, the victim must be watched closely for signs of returning anaphylaxis (shock), and another dose of epinephrine should be injected as often as every 15 minutes if needed. See page 20.

STROKE

A stroke is a life-threatening emergency! A stroke happens when a blood vessel in the brain bursts or is clogged by a blood clot or some

other particle. Because of this rupture or block-
age, part of the brain does not get the blood
flow it needs. Without oxygen, brain cells in
the affected area cannot function and die within
minutes.

WHAT TO LOOK FOR

The National Stroke Association gives these as
warning signs:

- Numbness, weakness, or paralysis of face,
  arm, or leg—especially on one side of the
  body
- Sudden blurred or decreased vision in one
  eye or both
- Difficulty speaking or understanding simple
  statements
- Loss of balance or coordination when combined with another warning sign
- Sudden unexplained headaches

About 10 percent of strokes are preceded by
"little strokes," known as transient ischemic attacks (TIAs). The usual symptoms of TIA are
brief episodes similar to those of stroke. More
than 75 percent of TIAs last less than 5 minutes.
The average is about a minute, although some
last several hours. Unlike stroke, when a TIA
is over, the victim returns to normal. Do not
ignore the symptoms. Get medical attention immediately.

WHAT TO DO

1 Check the ABCs.
2 Place the victim
in the proper position:
- *If the victim is con-
  scious,* raise the
  head and shoulders
  slightly to reduce

blood pressure on the
brain
- *If the victim is un-
  conscious,* place the
  victim on the side
  ("recovery posi-
  tion"). Positioning

on the side keeps the airway open and allows secretions to drain from the mouth.

3 DO NOT give anything to drink or eat since the throat may be paralyzed, which restricts swallowing.

4 Call the EMS immediately.

SUBSTANCE ABUSE

Substance abuse is the improper use of medical and nonmedical substances. These substances affect how the body functions. Substances are categorized according to their effects on the body: stimulants (i.e., cocaine, amphetamines), depressants (i.e., barbiturates, narcotics, alcohol, inhalants), and hallucinogens (i.e., LSD, PCP, mescaline).

WHAT TO DO

1 Check the ABCs.

2 Call the Poison Control Center for advice or call the EMS for help.

3 Try to find out what substance was taken, how much was taken, and when it was taken.

4 If person is vomiting, place on his or her side so that vomit will not be inhaled. If victim is vomiting, keep on the left side to reduce the likelihood of vomiting and inhalation of vomit. DO NOT let the person sleep on his or her back.

5 Provide reassurance and emotional support. DO NOT leave the person alone.

6 DO NOT try to handle a hostile or violent person by yourself. Find a safe place for yourself and call the police for help.

TICK EMBEDDED

Because of its painless bite, a tick can remain embedded for days without the victim ever knowing. Most tick bites are harmless, though ticks can carry serious diseases (i.e., Lyme disease, Rocky Mountain spotted fever).

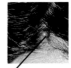

Tick embedded and engorged with victim's blood.

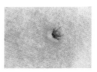

Tick embedded

WHAT TO DO

1 Pull off the tick using one of these methods:

- Use tweezers, or if you have to use your fingers, protect your skin by using a paper towel or disposable tissue or gloves.

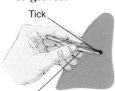

Tick

Remove a tick with tweezers

- Grasp the tick as close to the skin surface as possible and pull away from the skin with a steady pressure or lift the tick slightly upward and pull parallel to the skin until the tick detaches. DO NOT grab it at the rear of its body; the internal gut may rupture and the contents may be squeezed out, causing infection. DO NOT twist or jerk the tick; this may result in incomplete removal.

- DO NOT use the following popular methods of tick removal, which are not as effective:

    - Petroleum jelly
    - Fingernail polish
    - Rubbing alcohol
    - A blown-out hot match
    - Petroleum prod-

T

ucts (i.e., gasoline)

2 Wash the bite site with soap and water. Apply rubbing alcohol to disinfect the area.

3 Apply an ice pack to reduce pain.

4 Apply calamine lotion to relieve any itching. Keep the area clean.

5 Watch for signs of infection or unexplained symptoms (i.e., severe headache, fever, or rash), which may develop 3 to 10 days later. If symptoms appear, seek medical attention immediately.

Lyme disease symptoms:

- Varies from person to person
- Early stages: fatigue, fever, chills, weakness, distinctive rash, headaches, stiff necks, muscle or joint pains

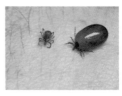

Deer ticks. Not engorged and blood engorged

- Later stages: one-sided paralysis, arthritis, meningitis, nerve or heart damage.

WOUNDS

WHAT TO DO

1 Protect yourself against disease by wearing disposable latex gloves. If disposable gloves are not available, use several layers of gauze pads, plastic wrap or bags, or even have the victim apply pressure with his or her hand.

Using your bare hand should be a last resort.

2 Expose the wound by removing or cutting the clothing to see where the blood is coming from.

3 Control bleeding (see page 18).

Cleaning Wounds

A victim's wound should be cleaned to help prevent infection. Wound cleaning may restart bleeding. If bleeding is severe, leave the pressure bandage in place until certain that bleeding has stopped.

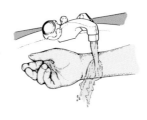

WHAT TO DO

1 Wash your hands with a vigorous scrubbing action, using soap and water. Wear disposable gloves.

2 Clean wound.
For a shallow wound:

- Wash the skin around the wound with soap and water. If a physician will not be seeing the wound or if you are in a remote setting, wash the skin around the wound and inside the wound with soap and water. DO NOT use hydrogen peroxide. It does not kill bacteria, and it adversely affects capillary blood flow and wound healing. DO NOT soak a wound to clean it.

- Run water (clean enough to drink) directly into the wound and allow it to run out. Irrigation with water needs pressure (i.e., faucet) for adequate tissue cleansing.

  For a wound with a high risk of infection (i.e., animal bite, very dirty, ragged, puncture), seek medical attention for wound cleaning. If you are in a remote setting, clean as best as you can.

3 Small objects not flushed out by irrigation can be removed with sterile tweezers. DO NOT clean large wounds or extremely dirty wounds; let emergency department personnel do the cleaning. DO NOT scrub a wound; scrubbing can bruise the tissue.

4 Cover the wound with a sterile dressing. DO NOT close the wound with tape (i.e., butterfly, steri-strips, etc.) because infection is more likely when bacteria are trapped in the wound. Keep the dressing clean and dry. When possible, use a nonstick dressing. For a shallow wound (one not needing stitches), an antibiotic ointment can be applied.

5 Change the dressing daily and more often if it gets wet or dirty.

W

Dressings and Bandages

DRESSINGS

A dressing covers a wound. Whenever possible, a dressing should be:

- Sterile. If a sterile dressing is not available use a clean cloth (i.e., handkerchief, wash-cloth, towel, etc.).
- Larger than the wound
- Thick, soft, and compressible so that pressure is evenly distributed over the wound
- Lint free

Types of Dressings

- Gauze pads. These are used for small wounds. They come in separately wrapped packages of various sizes (i.e., 2-inch by 2-inch; 4-inch by 4-inch) and are sterile, unless the package is broken. Some have a special coating to keep them from sticking to a burn or wound leaking fluids.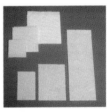
- Adhesive strips. These are used for small cuts and abrasions, and are a combination of both a sterile dressing and a bandage.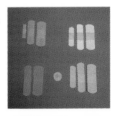
- Trauma (universal) dressings. These are made of thick, absorbent, sterile materials.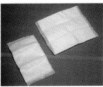

BANDAGES

A bandage holds a dressing in place over a wound or holds splints in place on the body. A bandage should be clean but need not be sterile. Bandages should be applied firmly enough to keep dressings and splints in place, but not so tight as to interfere with blood circulation.

Types of Bandages

1. Triangular bandage. A triangular bandage may be applied as:

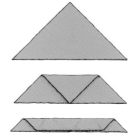

- Fully opened (not folded). Best used for an arm sling. Not recommended for holding a dressing in place since it does not apply sufficient pressure on the wound.

- Cravat (folded triangular). Used to hold splints in place, to apply pressure evenly over a dressing, or as a binder around the victim's body to stabilize an injured arm in an arm sling

2. Roller bandage. Roller bandages come in various widths, lengths, and types of material. For best results in different body areas, use

   1-inch width for finger
   2-inch width for ankle, elbow, wrist, hand
   3-inch width for ankle, elbow, arm
   4-inch width for knee, leg

- Self-adhering, conforming bandage. These come as rolls of slightly elastic, gauzelike material. They are available in various widths.

The self-adherent quality makes them easy to use.

- Gauze roller. These are cotton, nonelastic, and rigid. They come in various widths (1, 2, and 3 inches) and are usually 10 yards long.
- Elastic. These are used for compression bandages on sprains, strains, and contusions. They come in various widths. They are not usually applied over dressings covering a wound.

Applying a Roller Bandage

With a little ingenuity, roller bandages can be applied to almost any body part. Self-adhering, conforming roller bandages eliminate the need for many of the complicated bandaging techniques required with standard gauze roller, cravat, and triangular bandages.

- Spiral. For arms use 3-inch width; for legs use 4-inch width roller.
- Figure-8. This is a method of applying a roller bandage to hold dressings or to provide compression at or near a joint (i.e., ankle). The method involves continuous spiral loops of bandage, one up and one down, crossing each other to form an "8."

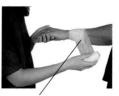
Two straight turns.

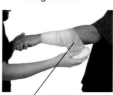
Spiral turns going up.

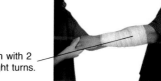
Finish with 2 straight turns.

Elbow or knee (3-inch for elbow; 4-inch for knee)

(1)

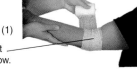
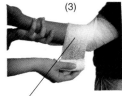

Make two straight turns around elbow.

(2)

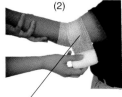

Bring bandage above joint.

(3)

Bring bandage below joint.

Hand (2-inch roller bandage)

(1)

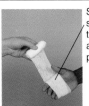

Start with 2 straight turns around palm.

(2)

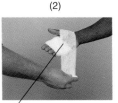

Diagonal turn across back of hand, around wrist, and back across palm.

Make several figure-8 turns overlapping ¾ of previous layer.

(3)

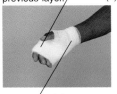

Make 2 straight turns at wrist and secure the end.

Ankle/foot (3-inch width) This wrapping is to hold a dressing or apply compression for treating a sprained ankle, not for supporting the ankle and foot during a sports activity

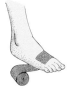

which involves additional maneuvers.

Secure a roller bandage with adhesive tape.

- Adhesive tape. Tape comes in rolls and in a variety of widths. It is often used to secure roller bandages and small dressings in place. For those allergic to adhesive tape, use paper tape or special dermatologic tape.

Triangular Bandage Slings

A triangular bandage used as a sling supports and protects the upper extremities. The sling is not a bandage but is used as a support for any injury to the shoulder or arm.

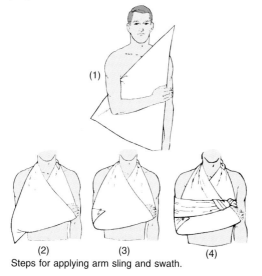

(1)

(2) (3) (4)

Steps for applying arm sling and swath.

Improvised slings can be made by:

- Placing the hand inside a buttoned jacket.
- Using a belt, necktie, or other clothing item looped around the neck and the injured arm.
- Turning up the lower edge of the victim's jacket or shirt over the injured arm and pinning it to the upper part of the jacket or shirt.
- Pinning a shirt sleeve to the shirt in the desired position.

Splinting Broken Bones and Dislocations

Applying a splint usually requires two people. One stabilizes and supports the injured limb while the other person applies the splint. Remember to check the **CSM** (circulation, sensation, movement) before applying a splint and periodically afterward.

Shoulder

Place an open triangular bandage between the forearm and chest. Bring the lower end over the forearm, under the armpit, and around the victim's back. Tie the lower end to the upper end. This stabilizes injuries to clavicle, most shoulder injuries, upper humerus fractures.

If the victim is holding his or her arm in a fixed position away from the chest wall, suspect a shoulder dislocation. Place a pillow or rolled blanket between the involved arm and the chest, to fill the space created, and then use cravats or roller bandage to secure the arm against the chest.

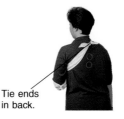

Injured shoulder or collarbone.

Bring one end over forearm and under armpit on injured side.

Tie ends in back.

Upper Arm (Humerus)

Place a splint (i.e., board, folded newspapers) along the outside of the arm. Place padding between the arm and the chest. Then apply a sling and cravat binder around the arm and body, using the chest wall also as a splint.

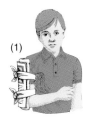
(1)

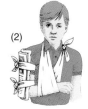
(2)

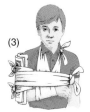
(3)

Elbow

Stabilize the elbow in the position found: if it is bent, splint it bent; if it is straight, splint it straight.

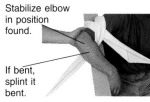

Stabilize elbow in position found.

If bent, splint it bent.

Completed splint for bent elbow.

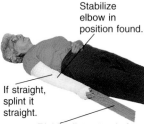

Stabilize elbow in position found.

If straight, splint it straight.

Rigid splint extends from hand to armpit.

Forearm

Whenever possible, place splints (i.e., boards, folded newspapers) on both sides of the injured part ("sandwich splint"). Place the arm in a sling

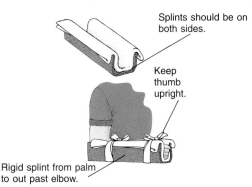

Splints should be on both sides.

Keep thumb upright.

Rigid splint from palm to out past elbow.

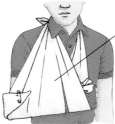

Arm sling (cravat binder not shown)

and secure with a cravat binder around the body. Keep the victim's thumb in an upright position to prevent rotation of the forearm bones.

Wrist, Hand, and Fingers

Stabilize the wrist and hand by attaching one splint (i.e., board, folded newspapers) that extends past the tip of the fingers to mid-forearm. Position the injured hand with bent fingers (looks like hand is holding a baseball) by placing a rolled pair of socks or cloths in the palm of the hand. Place the arm in a sling and cravat binder with the thumb in an upright position. Injured fingers may be taped together ("buddy taping"), with gauze separating the fingers.

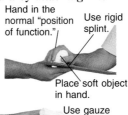

Hand in the normal "position of function."

Use rigid splint.

Place soft object in hand.

Use gauze roller bandage.

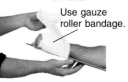

Overlap ½-¾ over previous layer.

Pelvis and Hip

Stabilize the victim as he or she is found; treat for shock (do not lift the legs); and wait for the EMS since these fractures require trained personnel and a long backboard (spine board). Pillows or other soft objects can be placed underneath the knees.

Thigh (Femur)

Stabilize the leg by placing folded blankets or pillows between the victim's legs for padding, and then tie the injured leg to the uninjured leg with several cravat bandages. Wait for the EMS because these fractures require trained personnel and specialized equipment.

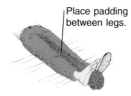
Place padding between legs.

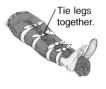
Tie legs together.

Knee

Stabilize an injured knee in the position found: If it is bent, splint it bent; if it is straight, splint it straight.

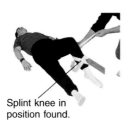
Splint knee in position found.

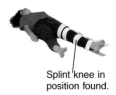
Splint knee in position found.

Lower Leg

Stabilize the lower leg with two boards extending from the middle of the thigh to the bottom of the foot, or tie the legs together as described for a broken thigh bone.

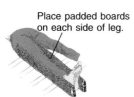
Place padded boards on each side of leg.

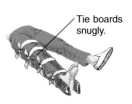
Tie boards snugly.

Ankle and Foot

Treat ankle and foot injuries with the **RICE** procedures (see page 108). See page 33 for information on ankle/foot in-

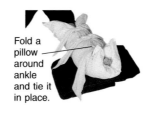

Fold a pillow around ankle and tie it in place.

juries. To stabilize an ankle further, wrap a pillow around the ankle and foot and tie with cravats.

Spine (Backbone)

DO NOT move the victim. Wait for the EMS because of their trained personnel and specialized equipment. See page 35 for more information.

Moving a Victim

A victim should not be moved until he or she has received all necessary first aid. If you move a victim, DO NOT make the injury worse. Move a victim from immediate danger, such as:

- A fire or danger of fire
- Explosives or other hazardous materials
- Impossibility of protecting the accident scene from hazards
- Impossibility of gaining access to other victims in a vehicle who need lifesaving care

SHOULDER DRAG

Use the shoulder drag when the victim is in danger and for short distances over a rough surface; stabilize victim's head with your forearms.

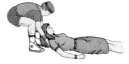

ONE-PERSON MOVES

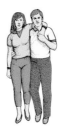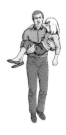

- *One person assist in helping victim to walk (human crutch):* If one leg is injured, help the victim to walk on the good leg while you support the injured side.
- *Cradle carry:* Used for children and lightweight adults who cannot walk.

- *Pack-strap carry:* Effective for a victim who is as big as or bigger than you.
- *Piggy-back carry:* Used when the victim cannot walk but can use the arms to hang onto to the rescuer.

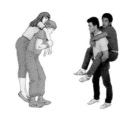

TWO-PERSON MOVES

- *Four-handed seat carry:* The easiest two-person carry when no equipment is available. The victim cannot walk but can use the arms to hang onto the two rescuers.
- *Extremity carry*

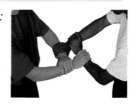

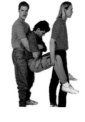

- *Chair carry:* Use a sturdy chair that can hold the victim's weight.

Appendix A

RICE Procedures for Muscle, Joint, and Bone Injuries

The acronym **RICE** is used to remember the first aid procedures for contusions (bruises), strains, sprains, dislocations, and fractures.

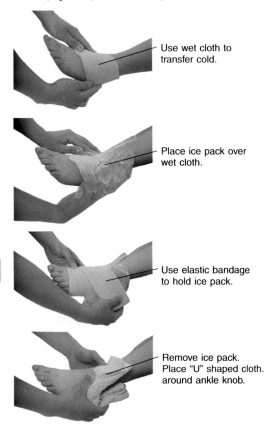

Use wet cloth to transfer cold.

Place ice pack over wet cloth.

Use elastic bandage to hold ice pack.

Remove ice pack. Place "U" shaped cloth. around ankle knob.

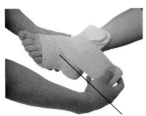

Use elastic bandage to
hold "U" shaped cloth.

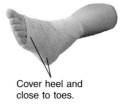

Cover heel and
close to toes.

R = *Rest*

The first initial, R, stands for rest. This means
that the victim should stop moving the injured
part. Any injury heals faster if rested.

I = *Ice*

The second initial, I, stands for ice. An ice pack
should be applied immediately to the injured
area for 20 to 30 minutes and every 2 to 3 hours
during the next 24 to 48 hours. The skin being
treated with cold passes through four stages—
cold, burning, aching, and numbness. When it
becomes numb, remove the ice pack. This usually takes 20 to 30 minutes. After removing an
ice pack, keep the part compressed with an elastic bandage and elevated (techniques covered
later).

C = *Compression*

The third initial, C, stands for compression.
Compression applied by an elastic bandage over
the injury can squeeze some fluid and debris out
of the injury site. Elastic bandages come in various widths. For best results in different body
areas, use:

2-inch width for ankle, hand, wrist
3-inch width for ankle, elbow, arm
4-inch width for knee, thigh, leg

Start the elastic bandage several inches below the injury and wrap in an upward, overlapping (about ¾ its width) spiral, starting with

even and somewhat tight pressure, then gradually wrapping looser above the injury.

The victim should wear the elastic bandage continuously for the first 18 to 24 hours. Remove the elastic bandage while applying cold 3 to 4 times daily, and replace it after each cold application. At night, have the victim loosen, but not remove, the elastic bandage.

For an ankle injury, place one of the victim's socks or a towel shaped like a "horseshoe" on the injured side and around the ankle knob next to the skin and under the elastic bandage. This compresses the soft tissues rather than just the bones and tendon.

For a bruised or strained muscle, place a pad over the injury and under the elastic bandage for compression.

E = *Elevation*

The fourth initial, E, stands for elevation. Elevating the injured area in combination with ice and compression limits circulation to that area and, therefore, helps limit internal bleeding and swelling.

Whenever possible, raise the injured part above the level of the heart for the first 24 hours after an injury.

Appendix B

First Aid Supplies

Many injuries and sudden illnesses require first aid supplies. Supplies should be customized to include those items likely to be used on a regular basis.

The list below includes nonprescriptive (over-the-counter) medications. Some drug products lose their potency over time, especially after they are opened. Other drugs change in consistency. Buying the large "family size" of a product infrequently used may seem like a bargain, but it is poor economy if the product has to be thrown out before the contents are used. Medications have an expiration date.

Keep all medicines out of the reach of children.

Keep your first aid supplies in either a fishing tackle box or a tool box. Boxes with an O-ring gasket around the cover are dustproof and waterproof.

EQUIPMENT

Scissors
- Regular
- Bandage (blunt-tip prevents injury while cutting next to skin)
- EMT shears (cuts through metal, leather, heavy clothing)

Tweezers (remove splinters, ticks, small objects from wound)

Pocket knife, folding

Disposable gloves, latex (protection against disease)

Mouth-to-barrier device, face mask with 1-way valve or face shield (protection against disease during rescue breathing)

Thermometer (measure body temperature)

Penlight; two types: replaceable battery or disposable

Light stick

Resealable plastic bags, pint and quart (ice pack, irrigating wound, amputation care)

Ice bag (ice pack)

Cotton-tipped swabs (remove small objects from eye, to evert eyelid, to apply ointment)

Extractor, from Sawyer Products (suction removes snakebite venom)

SAM splint (stabilize almost any part of the body)

Emergency blanket (protects victim from weather)

Safety pins, size 3 (hold bandages in place, improvising slings)

BANDAGE AND DRESSING MATERIALS

Gauze pads, 2-inch by 2-inch, 3-inch by 3-inch, 4-inch by 4-inch (stop bleeding and cover wound)

Non-stick pads, 2-inch by 3-inch, 3-inch by 4-inch (cover abrasions and small burns)

Adhesive strip bandages, various sizes and materials (cover small wounds)

Trauma dressings, 5-inch by 9-inch, 8-inch by 10-inch (cover large wounds)

Gauze roller bandages, 1-inch, 2-inch (hold dressings in place)

Conforming, self-adhering roller bandages, 2-inch, 3-inch, 4½-inch (hold dressings in place)

Elastic roller bandages, 2-inch, 3-inch, 4-inch, 6-inch (compression on sprains and strains)

Adhesive tape, 1/2-inch or 1-inch (hold dressings in place; secure end of roller bandages)

Hypoallergenic paper tape (hold dressings in place; prevents skin reactions)

Waterproof tape (hold dressings in place)

Knuckle bandages

Fingertip strips

Eye pads

Triangular bandages (arm sling and forms cravat bandages for holding splints in place)

Moleskin and molefoam (blister prevention and care)

Duct tape, roll (blister prevention, holding splints in place)

OINTMENTS AND TOPICALS

Antiseptic towelettes (cleaning skin around wounds and hands)

Alcohol prep pads (cleaning skin around wounds)

Antibiotic ointment (minor cuts, abrasions, burns)

Hydrocortisone cream, 1 percent (skin irritation and itching)

Antifungal cream

Calamine lotion (anti-itch and drying agent for poison ivy, oak, sumac, and skin rashes)

Sting relief swabs (relieve pain from insect bites and stings)

Instant ice pack (use when ice is not available)

Spenco Second Skin Pads (blister care)

Aloe vera gel, 100 percent (minor burns, frostbite)

Sun screen (SPF 15)

Lip balm with sunscreen (protects lips)

Insect repellant, containing less than 30 percent DEET

OVER-THE-COUNTER INTERNAL MEDICATIONS

Aspirin (for pain, swelling, and fever)
Ibuprofen (for pain, swelling, and fever)
Acetaminophen (for pain)
Antihistamine (for allergy)
Decongestant, tablets and nasal spray
Antacid (for gas)
Antidiarrhea, antinausea/vomiting
Anticonstipation
Anti-motion sickness
Glucose paste (for insulin reaction)
Oil of cloves (for toothache)
Activated charcoal, pre-mixed liquid (for swallowed poisoning)
Ipecac syrup (use only when medical authority directs for swallowed poisoning)
Cough suppressant
Powered electrolyte drink mix (for heat stress)

MISCELLANEOUS

Pencil and small notebook (for recording information and sending messages) and the *National Safety Council* First Aid Pocket Guide.

Emergency Index

Abdominal injuries, 29
Abdominal pain, 30
Allergic reaction, 20
Amputations, 30
Animal bites, 31
Ankle/foot injuries, 33
Asthma, 34

Back/neck injuries, 35
Bleeding, 18
Blisters, 37
Breathing, rescue, 8
Broken bone, 39
Bruise, 41
Burns, heat/thermal, 42

Chemical exposure, 24
Chest injuries, 46
Chest pain, 48
Choking, 10
CPR, 8

Dental/mouth injuries, 49
Diabetic Emergencies, 27, 51
Dislocation, 52

Electrocution, 53
Eye injuries, 53

Fainting, 57
Finger/toe injuries, 58
Frostbite, 61

Head injuries, 62
Heart attack, 21
Heat illnesses, 23, 66
Help, getting, 4
Hyperventilation, 68
Hypothermia, 69

Muscle injuries, 72

Nose injuries, 72

Poison, swallowed/ingested, 74
Poison ivy, oak, and sumac, 75

Seizures, 78
Shock, 79
Snakebites, 81
Spider bites and scorpion stings, 84
Stings, insect, 87
Stroke, 88
Substance abuse, 90

Tick embedded, 91

Wounds, 92